endorsements

Menopause is one of the last taboo topics. Women dread trading hot sex for hot flashes. But now, in this gloriously honest conversation, Brouk and Stockwell invite us to explore new possibilities for turning the dreaded 'change of life' into a personal transformation.

Sally Hogshead, New York Times bestselling author and creator of How to Fascinate®

Open and candid conversations about the incredible wisdom that unveils as women move into menopause, how genius! When I was younger, I vowed to shift the idea of menopause from dread and embarrassment into empowerment and grace. I found that type of support in this book. The courageous authors Tricia Brouk and Alexandra Stockwell, MD, created the perfect intimate container for all of us to converse and connect. The Invitation is a new movement; I can't wait to see it unfold.

Mari Carmen Pizarro Founder of The International Leadership Academy for Women

This is like talking to your best friend about Menopause and exploring everything that no one dared to discuss before. It's so needed!

Alexandra Dean, Documentary director

The Invitation delivers. From time to time, we all need permission to explore life's subjects with complete freedom. Freedom for us, freedom for those we love, freedom for our community. This last freedom is most important for future generations to thrive. To be more open, more prepared. And this preparation is our gift, our legacy. It's the dream of all authors, creators, and those among us who bring new life to words, ideas, and feelings. And that is the message inside *The Invitation.*

Menopause can be daunting, or it can be a beautiful chance to grow together, moving past old paradigms to a new way of loving. Our relationships, especially our loving, intimate relationships, can be powerful foundations for growth and emotional evolution, but only if we feel safe and unafraid to go deeper with ourselves and our partners. Tricia Brouk and Alexandra Stockwell come together to share details about life, love, and connection in a way that gives each of us permission to have these life-affirming conversations.

Two heart-centered women have given You a beautiful gift. An Invitation.

As men, we often feel left out of certain conversations. We think the dark corners are reserved for "women only." And this book shines a light on those areas. It's time to go into the dark to find the light inside you and your partner. I'm so grateful to have received *The Invitation.* Now it's your turn to accept it.

Rick Gabrielly, Co-Author, The Currency of Connection

In *The Invitation*, Tricia Brouk and Alexandra Stockwell, MD, fearlessly and transparently address menopause with grace and compassion. This groundbreaking book offers valuable insights, practical advice, and empowering perspectives. It demystifies menopause, fosters open conversations, and empowers women to embrace this transformative journey with resilience and joy.

The collaborative effort of Brouk and Stockwell adds a unique perspective to the book. Their combined expertise and complementary insights provide a holistic understanding of menopause, addressing both the physical and emotional aspects with equal care.

Steph Tuss CEO of Life is Now Inc.

What a beautiful shift in perspective! While I had been thinking of menopause as an irritation of womanhood, I now see it as an initiation into wisdomhood. This book truly is an invitation to cross the threshold, shed our old skin, and migrate from one phase of our life into a new beautiful version of ourselves.

Tanya Dalton, Best-selling author of The Joy of Missing Out and Keynote Speaker

Vulnerable conversations with so much valuable information. Tricia and Alexandra's journey will resonate with so many. Come for the insights, stay for the connection. A must read.

Dr. Meghna Dassani - Functional and Sleep Apnea Dentist

The Invitation is a powerful and intimate conversation between two women who deeply care about each other's voices and every woman's well-being. The book is a poignant, playful, and honest conversation about being a woman experiencing what menopause means to their physical selves, emotional selves and spiritual selves. Any woman or their partner will benefit from being invited into this tender conversation.

Susan Winter, Bestselling Author/Relationship Expert

As a woman in her 30s who just had a baby, I don't exactly have menopause on the brain, so I didn't know what to expect from this book. But being privy to this vulnerable and insightful dialogue between these two brave women has been transformational. I feel a sense of calm and gratitude for being given the gift of knowledge and an understanding of what's down the road for me. And even more importantly, an even greater appreciation and admiration for my body (which I didn't think was possible).

Emily Williams, Founder and CEO of I Heart My Life

the
invitation

the invitation

VITAL
CONVERSATIONS
ABOUT
MENOPAUSE

TRICIA BROUK AND
ALEXANDRA STOCKWELL, MD

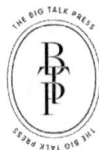

THE BIG TALK PRESS

the invitation

VITAL CONVERSATIONS ABOUT MENOPAUSE

TRICIA BROUK AND ALEXANDRA STOCKWELL, MD

Visit the authors' websites at:
triciabrouk.com
alexandrastockwell.com

Published and distributed by Big Talk Press
New York, USA
thebigtalkpress.com

Library of Congress Control Number: 2023908559
Brouk, Tricia & Stockwell, Alexandra
The Invitation: Vital Conversations About Menopause
ISBN: 978-1-960553-00-3 Paperback

For women, and their partners, who want to live fully with power, joy, elegance, and connection.

This book is intended to inspire conversations among readers and their friends and family. It is not intended to diagnose or treat menopause and should not be used to do so.

CONTENTS

INTRODUCTION

In October of 2022, I opened my home to my dear friend and colleague, Dr. Alexandra Stockwell, so that we could sit down and co-author a book. The whole experience was better and more fulfilling than we could have imagined.

Nine months prior, I had sent her a text that cryptically said, "I'd love to discuss something with you. When can you get on a call?" She responded right away, and we scheduled a time to speak.

On our call, I shared I wanted to write a book about menopause and that I wanted her to be my co-author. Giddy and greatly surprised, she right away said an initial "yes" while asking for some time to consider the unexpected invitation. A few days later, when she arrived at a full yes, we began co-creating.

We first focused on our process of how we would birth this book. Then we articulated our vision: who the book would be for, the contribution it would make, and whom we would involve in creating it. We also acknowledged that a book about menopause is not something that fits into either one of our business models or brands. We talked that through and embraced it, making clear that our reasons for writing together were feeling strongly about the topic and looking forward to the collaboration we were embarking on.

We also decided that the book writing process would be easy and generative. We are both successful entrepreneurs who have already written books, and we wanted this process to be luxurious.

Alexandra flew to New York City from San Francisco, leaving her family for four days. My husband, Joe, left our apartment to allow Alexandra and me privacy from 9am to 5pm on the two days we would be working together. In advance of the first work session, I prepared our home with bouquets of yellow roses and pale pink roses to bring in feminine and sacral womb energy. I lit a special candle labeled "written in the stars." We had essential oils to enhance creativity, and I rang a bell to open the sacred portal before we began. I provided nourishing foods like blueberries, raw almonds, and dark organic chocolate throughout the weekend. We wrote letters of intention to one another ahead of time and began by reading them aloud.

Part of our desire for ease included deciding that what we shared with each other during those two days would provide the content that would become the book. We had arranged ahead of time for the incredible Barrie Cole, a writer and playwright, to support us. She would be developing and transforming our conversations into a book by reading, rereading, and then assiduously shaping hours of transcripts into something tangible, accessible, relatable, and real.

During the two days we spent together, we interviewed Pat Duckworth, a total badass in the UK whose platform is menopause in the workplace. We had never met her before and found her generous, articulate, deep, and compelling.

It was important for us to capture the voices of women in menopause who are having the experience of, well, being intensely pissed off. Alexandra and I are more vital, energetic, and powerful than ever during menopause; however, that's definitely not the case for everyone. So we interviewed three incredible women I admire who are having a really challenging time during their menopause journey. What they shared about the healthcare system is also an important part of this conversation.

We addressed all the things we could think of so that our weekend together would feel complete, including a one-hour photo shoot with Micah Joel, so we'd have photos for the book and wouldn't have to schedule another time to capture them.

The two days we spent together in recorded conversations were sublime, creative, expansive, vulnerable, and fun. I knew we would be able to accomplish something special and that I would be different because of it. But I didn't anticipate how much I would miss Alexandra when she left. There was a real tenderness to our time together and in the quality of connection that emerged through speaking about menopause. A sisterhood was created, and it's available for all women through reading this book– a book that invites the reader to be in conversation with us, themselves, their families, and their communities.

We hope this will be your invitation to embrace your body, your season of life, and your journey with menopause (as well as a guide for others who support you in doing so).

Tricia Brouk

New York City

chapter 1

THE BEGINNING
BEFORE THE BEGINNING

Tricia: Alexandra, I'm recording everything. I want to be able to hear everything we say from the moment we first embrace.

Alexandra: Wow, okay. Oh my God, it's so good to see you. You look beautiful. But I have to tell you that I'm nervous. I'm really, really nervous.

Tricia: I love how nervous you are. May I take your coat?

Alexandra: Yes, thank you.

Tricia: Good. So this is my home.

Alexandra: Oh, my! It's where everything happens!

Tricia: Yes. Yes. Yes.

Alexandra: This moment reminds me a bit of when I was in medical school, my second year. I lived with two Muslim women, one of them wore a hijab, and one didn't. The one who wore a hijab, after we had developed a very deep friendship, invited me into her room, and her hijab was off.

Tricia: That's so intimate.

Alexandra: It was extraordinarily intimate. Having had that experience, I forever have a different relationship with what it is to wear a hijab. Anyway, I mention that because it feels like this is an equivalent experience because I've seen your backdrop online numerous times, but now I see the whole room in three dimensions. I feel vulnerable as if you're revealing something personal in a way that made me think of my Muslim friend.

Tricia: Oh, yes.

Alexandra: Your home is wonderful.

Tricia: Thank you. This is Esther, my Jade money tree, whom I love and adore. This is Bella, one of our cat daughters. She likes the top of her head rubbed, and she's very shy.

Alexandra: She's such a lion. Her physique is remarkable.

Tricia: Oh, she's definitely a lion.

Alexandra: So beautiful.

Tricia: Our other furry daughter, Lola, is in the other room. You'll meet her in a second. They have such different personalities. It's amazing.

Alexandra: So sweet. I love the sound of their purring.

Tricia: Out this window over here are the Alvin Ailey Dance Studios. Every single day, looking out my window, I get to watch dreams being realized. It brings me so much joy.

Alexandra: Wow. I love that you stay connected to the dance world in this way.

Tricia: Lola is 18 years old and has arthritis, but we still want her to enjoy her independence, so now we have these little cat staircases everywhere.

Alexandra: They are very elegant.

Tricia: Here's a photo…You've heard me talk about my dance competition years. I was thirteen years old when this was taken.

Alexandra: Wow, Tricia. Look at you!

Tricia: Buck teeth and big ears.

Alexandra: That's not what I see when I look at this. "Buck teeth and big ears" would never have come to my mind. I see "tenacity and presence."

Tricia: Really? Thank you. Here's a series from my first solo show called Dining Alone. The photoshoot was super fun.

Alexandra: You look magnificent. It's really enjoyable for me to see all of this and to get to know you in new ways.

Tricia: These photos are from when we adopted Bella. My husband, Joe, and I drove all the way from New York to South Carolina to get her.

This picture is from when we went to the Jean-George restaurant for our anniversary. The server asked us if we would like a tour of the kitchen, and, well, of course, we did! Joe asked if he could take a photo, and the entire kitchen staff stopped what they were doing to take a photograph with us.

Alexandra: Wow. It looks like something taken from a film.

Tricia: We laughed for a good 20 minutes because when a Michelin Star Restaurant stops to take a pic, it's magical.

Over here is our piano. Joe asked for piano lessons for his birthday last November–he loved them so much that he needed to get a piano. Now we sing and play the piano together at the end of the night. It's the most joyous thing ever. It's really the best.

Alexandra: That's fantastic.

Tricia: It really is.

Alexandra: I still can't get over the view here. I can see the whole skyline.

Tricia: I love it. In our former apartment, we didn't have nice windows or light.

Alexandra: This must be such a change. Remind me when you moved here…

Tricia: We've been here for three and a half years. During the pandemic, Joe thanked me every single day. Everything would have been so much harder in the other space. Here we look at the most gorgeous New York City skyline. I love it.

You're seeing everything at a certain time of day. It's not actually so clear right now, but if you look closely, you can see that this building reflects hugs and kisses. You can see Xs and Os. It's slightly past when they're at their peak, but clear or not, I love seeing the hugs and kisses reflected there.

Alexandra: I see them. How wonderful!

Tricia: I love having you here. I mean, this is the view that I talk about all the time on social media. I call these windows THE wraparound windows.

Alexandra: I don't think I've ever seen a New York apartment like this. I'm just so happy to be here.

chapter 2

THE BEGINNING

Tricia: Shall we begin?

Alexandra: Yes.

Tricia: I would love to read my letter aloud to you just because it feels important. Is that okay with you?

Alexandra: Yes!

Tricia: I love it. Okay, here we go! I'm so glad we decided to write these letters to each other. The reason I'm reading it again is so I can be reminded of how I felt when I wrote it.

Dear Alexandra,

This is a ceremony of sacred sharing and creation.

I come to this process with devotion and vulnerability, knowing that we are meant to be doing this together. In this way, I would like to acknowledge all women—through talking about menopause so openly, we offer freedom, self-love, and acceptance. Menopause does not have the power to suppress our creativity. It is our natural, aligned state. So many women have an energy of trauma around menopause before they ever even enter into it. I'd love to remove the stigma from menopause and free women experiencing it from imposed worry, fear, or shame.

We have an opportunity to help heal the shame of others by fully embracing and embodying ourselves as women who are living life full out and full on. The womb is a creative portal. This creation, this conversation, and the book we are birthing is coming from our wombs.

I will be creating an environment of love, joy, and comfort. This space will have yellow roses, the sacred womb color, as well as pale pink for femininity. I will have essential oils and candles. It is an altar of sorts. We'll have water, iced teas, and healthy snacks, and I'll provide us with a nourishing lunch. I would love to open and close our container with the ringing of a bell. And we'll be able to go outside anytime, to be with nature too.

So Much Big Love,

Tricia

Alexandra:

Dear Tricia,

I wholeheartedly receive and affirm this letter of intention. I am writing from the airport in San Francisco. I am orienting myself to the journey both literally and figuratively, and I am doing so with humility, enthusiasm, and openness.

I'm aware that there is a wave of intention and attention on menopause that we are a part of, as this very weekend, the inaugural menopause summit is taking place in Manhattan. The stated goal of the summit is "Creating a movement that ends the stigma and starts conversations about this very natural, yet little discussed phase of life." Through our conversations, which will become a book, we are contributing to this emerging movement.

There's a way in which this book isn't only about menopause; it's about being a human being. I am excited for that to emerge while we focus on matters of menopause.

I love your passion and the stand you express and embody in any project you take on. I, too, stand for certain things in the world and want to honor and express that in any project I participate in.

As we've discussed, this book is about menopause, and neither one of us focuses on menopause in our respective business models. However, having said that a few times, I have begun to see that maybe it's not as simple as that. I mean, it's true at the level of marketing and strategy that neither of us focuses on menopause in our business, but it's not true at the level of mission. The deeper we get into creating this book, the more evident it is becoming that this project is deeply aligned with the truth each of us is dedicated to, both personally and professionally. For this book on menopause is also a book about women's voices (your expertise), and it's also a book about embodiment, pleasure, and connection with others (my expertise).

As we embark on our weekend together, I really love that we have clarity of intention, a felt sense of the relevance of collaboration, and openness to where this journey will lead us. There's a welcome freedom in going deep on a project that doesn't have a particular role in either of our business models, which I'm very much enjoying.

I appreciate you opening your home and creating a sacred space to support and attune our process. I also love that all elements of our process are rooted in a harmonious blending of what each of us brings to the table, with a fertile sense of creating something together. I am deeply honored to be here with you.

Love,

Alexandra

Tricia: I have been anticipating this date with such excitement. I've never done this before, and doing new things is super fun for me. Also, it feels so comfortable.

I notice that having a creative process that is not burdened with an outcome feels so expansive.

Alexandra: Yes, one of my personal riches in our process is how magnificent it feels absent a clear destination, a clear goal to meet. It's all about the process and responding to what emerges between us.

Tricia: Absolutely. I like our clearly unclear, meandering compass.

Here we go. We are officially beginning.

Alexandra: Yes, it's time.

Tricia: Alright, we are in New York City, where I've lived for more than thirty years. I'm definitely a New Yorker, and I also identify as a Midwesterner. What I mean by that is that I'm extremely hardworking, and I'm fearless. That's probably the dancer in me as well. I'm also a very trustworthy person. When I say I'll do something, I follow through. My word is everything.

I turned fifty in August 2020. I had been on birth control pills my entire adult life because I never wanted kids, and I never wanted to accidentally get pregnant. This statement may be controversial to some of our readers, and it's my hope that, as humans, we have grace and acceptance for one another while navigating through this conversation. In 2020, my gynecologist said, "Let's keep you on the pill for another year. There's a lot going on in the world right now. Not knowing what your body is going to do after we take you off hormones is probably not the best idea. I think you should wait another year."

So a year later, in July of 2021, on July first actually, I went off the pill. Everyone was telling me, "You know, Tricia, now you're going to see what is really going on with your body." The tone of their voices suggested to me that some scary, horrible things would be revealed. I proceeded anyway and purchased a diva cup in case I had my period. And I waited for my period. I waited, waited, and waited some more, and I never had a period. After a full year of waiting, I realized I had entered menopause. I was so happy not to have a period. It was not ambiguous for me at all.

Alexandra: This is amazing to hear in such clear terms.

Tricia: After two months, I began having serious hot flashes at night, not during the day, but in bed at night. I would wake up and feel this powerful energy in my body. I would acknowledge it, saying to myself, "Wow, it's so incredible that my body is having this experience." I would thank my body for being alive and for the privilege of being in this moment in time.

A few weeks later, I started to have hot flashes during the day and began taking off one piece of clothing at a time. I came to terms with the fact that turtlenecks may no longer be a part of my wardrobe!

The doctors and practitioners I consulted said all kinds of things that seemed strange to me. My whole medical journey is a big conversation that we have to spend more time on, but for now, I'll share what one doctor said, "You should go on all these hormones immediately. How you are alive is beyond me. How are you walking? Your hormones are entirely gone. You have no hormones." I thought, "Really? That sounds odd." So I sought a second opinion, then a third opinion. A naturopath said to me, "Your hormones are perfect. You don't need to do anything. I've never seen anybody so healthy or so perfectly aligned. Yes, you're in menopause, but there's no reason to do anything." That's when I decided I would turn inward and adjust my own experience in relation to the hot flashes.

I decided to use hypnotherapy to turn the dials of what my body needed. When I made that decision, and it was a decision with a capital D because I was dead serious about taking complete charge of my body and my health, I became more vibrant and much healthier. Sleeping, sex, the hot flashes, my energy level, everything just became exactly the way it was supposed to be. I have never felt more empowered, which is why I reached out to you about writing a book about menopause.

You've heard me say this before, but you're the only person that came to mind. If you had said, "No," I don't think I'd be doing this project. There was no other person I wanted to co-create this with. I knew I could be completely vulnerable with you.

I am nervous about being so honest and open about this. I haven't talked about any of this on social media or publicly at all. But I want to, and I want to with you, because it's important. It's really, really important.

Alexandra: I have some questions. I'd like you to expand on your experience early on in your process by describing in more detail what happened before you decided to go within and take control using hypnotherapy. How did you make that choice? What exactly were you going to the doctor for when you were getting all the opinions before going to the naturopath? What were you hoping to get from the doctor, such that you decided you no longer wanted it and would manage your symptoms on your own instead?

Tricia: Well, I went to the doctor initially because I wanted to have extensive blood work done in order to understand exactly where I was in the process of menopause.

Alexandra: Why was it important to identify where you were in the process?

Tricia: Great question. I think it was because I was determined not to have anything change. When I went off the pill, I thought, "Well, I've been manipulating my hormones my entire life anyway, so I might as well just keep manipulating my hormones." I told my OBGYN that I wanted the cream, the patch, everything. I said, "Please, give it all to me. I don't want to have any gap between when I go off the pill and when I go on the new stuff. I want to go right into it without missing a beat."

Alexandra: This makes me think of a widespread phenomenon that I encounter in my work as a relationship and intimacy coach. People assume in the course of their lifetime, as they age, they will advance and evolve both professionally and personally. As the years pass, they expect to earn more money and receive more accolades. They will be promoted and live in bigger homes (until they start downsizing after retirement). Growth and improvement are assumed in many areas. Except when it comes to sex.

When it comes to sex, many people have an idea that it's ideal to keep things as they were when they were twenty-five or thirty years old. When sex doesn't remain that way, frustrations mount. Some couples let it go and stop having sex altogether. What is unfortunate about this mindset is that it results in missing out on the sex that's available in our forties, fifties, sixties, and seventies and for the rest of our lives. It's the same with having children. Parents want their lives to be the way they were before having kids and often try in vain, becoming very frustrated at being unable to make it so. But sameness is not in the nature of growth and evolution. And sex and sensuality are definitely an arena of growth and evolution.

Getting back to what you said, it sounds like you initially wanted everything to stay the same, and in that sense, you wanted to avoid being held back by menopause. It's understandable, but it means you were essentially looking to deny its impact.

Wanting everything to stay the same is a fantasy that I think most people participate in, to some extent, either consciously or unconsciously, at different points in their lives.

Tricia: Oh, completely. I didn't think of it through that lens at the time, but I can see now that I was consciously trying not to evolve!

Alexandra: To me, that seems to go against your character and contrasts with how you approach every other part of your life.

Tricia: Yes, I realized I was not embracing possibility or potential, and that did not align with who I am or my beliefs!

I was driven by fear because I saw what my mother went through and how much she suffered. I knew that I needed to experience menopause in a different way than she had, both because of who I am and also because I had much more conscious awareness than she had had. I didn't want to feel like a victim of something; I wanted to participate. But I didn't know what would happen, and the specter of the unknown resulted in me getting in my own way.

Alexandra: I get it, and I really want to emphasize that. You and I are ambitious women who don't even question whether our lives will be meaningful. We are used to questioning the status quo in many areas of life; in fact, there's no other part of life that we've approached in this way. When it comes to menopause, why would we try to avoid evolution?

Tricia: Right! That's such a significant observation which provides yet another reason why it's so important to have this conversation. Hopefully, anyone who's reading this won't make the mistakes I made.

Alexandra: I love that outlook. In fact, this exchange makes me want to play with our title. It could be something like *Menopause: A Woman's Evolution.* I'm not attached to it, but I'd love for the title to point to something about the quality of evolving that's available during menopause.

Tricia: Yes, I like that. Menopause really is an evolution.

I'm fifty-two years old. I'm glad I decided not to listen to the first doctor who told me that my hormones were non-existent and I should take everything medicine had to offer me. Or my gynecologist, who said, "Why don't you just wait and see what happens?" "What do you mean, wait and see what happens? Things could go downhill really fast!"

I needed to summon the courage to chart my own course with minimal guidance outside myself.

Alexandra: Right, right. Let's go back to where you wanted to achieve as little change as possible. So you sought out and received multiple opinions from various doctors. Was it significant for you to then see a naturopath, or was that typical for you? I'm wondering if seeing a naturopath was previously uncharted territory?

Tricia: Well, ironically, the first doctor I saw was also a naturopath. He was the person who said that I needed to go on hormones. After hearing that, I called my OB-GYN and told her about my plan. "I'm going to go on all these hormones. I'm going to do all this stuff. I'm going to be amazing. It's all going to be great." She's the one who said, "Why?" I responded, "Well because I'm supposed to. It seems I need to." "How do you know that? You just went off the pill." I said, "Okay, you're right. I don't know that."

That's when I went to see another naturopath who happens to be a woman. It's very interesting because in between the first naturopath, my OB-GYN, and the second naturopath, I made the decision to go inside and recalibrate my hormone dials. I put this intention into my morning routine, and through my daily practice, I was able to stop my own hot flashes. That's when I realized, or remembered, that I can attract or create whatever I desire.

What in the world had me think for one second that I couldn't do that with my body? I took back my power and decided to go to a second naturopath to see if anything had changed with my blood work. Interestingly, nothing had really changed, but the second naturopath interpreted my test results differently. When I heard her interpretation, it gave me permission to be totally fine without doing anything, medically speaking.

I decided my medicine would be my meditation and hypnotherapy practices. That's what I did, and that period of time empowered me more than I ever could have imagined. I'm 100 percent free from all synthetic hormones now.

Alexandra: You both stopped the pill and also took no other hormones?

Tricia: Right. This was the very first time in my adulthood I wasn't taking hormones. Essentially, I had been manipulating my hormones, with the desired outcome of never getting pregnant, well before any hormonal shifts from menopause. So now, not only am I not able to get pregnant, but I'm also not on any hormone replacement or hormonal birth control. It's an amazing experience. The whole situation is brand new to me.

Alexandra: What have you noticed so far?

Tricia: I've noticed that I am more vibrant and more vital. I've always been rather vital and vibrant, but now, there is something about my body that I love even more. I love living in my skin, in this body of mine. I feel sexier, more beautiful, smarter, I feel more capable. I don't care what other people think. I really never have, but it's more solidified now.

Another change I have noticed is a new sense of not being attached to specific outcomes. I know that if I want something to happen and it doesn't, then something else will. I would never have felt that way, even just two years ago. It feels healthy to have much more detachment. I suppose I don't know if these changes are related to hormones necessarily. But I am sure that I had a kind of forceful energy before, an "I need to make this happen" energy. That is falling away.

In some ways, I am like a young girl, a female being who is not yet a woman. Young girls passionately care about what happens without getting distracted by all the various considerations. Tricia, the woman, is clear and strong in that same way. Worry isn't running the show, and to some degree, it was before. Now, it's very clear–I have my point of view. I trust it. There's not much more to say about it.

I have evolved and love that I have become trustworthy for my vision, my values, and myself. I access more joy and love. Truly, I have never been happier, and I am in the thick of menopause, the same full-blown menopause dreaded by so many.

Notice that choice of language? Why did I choose to use the phrase "full-blown"? Even the words I use are more expressive. I find my whole menopausal landscape surprising and delightful.

Alexandra: I'm sure some people would not believe menopause, the way you're experiencing it, is even possible. Yet, here you are, having your authentic experience.

Tricia: I'm speaking the truth. Sharing my reality. Using my voice.

chapter 3

MAKING SENSE
OF SYMPTOMS

Alexandra: Shall I tell my story now?

Tricia: I would love to hear your story.

Alexandra: I'll begin by saying that, somewhere along the way, I learned that women tend to go through menopause the same way their mothers go through menopause. I don't know how my mother went through menopause, although I wish I did, and it has left me feeling like the ground is a bit wobbly on this subject. As you and I have considered how invisible and rarely discussed menopause is, I've often thought of my mother and my lack of information.

My mother died just after she turned sixty. At the time, I was thirty-four. She died from breast cancer, and we knew she was terminal for a few months beforehand. This meant there was time to discuss all kinds of things that wouldn't have come up if we hadn't been anticipating her death. However, with all the things I asked her (I asked so very many questions before she died), not once did it occur to me to ask her about menopause. It just never crossed my mind. If it had, I definitely would have asked.

What this means is that anticipating my own menopause, I felt like I was in the dark. No particular expectations, no relevant information specific to me and my maternal line. No sense of the challenges or the ways to successfully navigate them. No idea if my mother had suffered. No idea if it never came up because there wasn't much to say. "In the dark" is the best description of how I felt anticipating my own menopause.

The only information I have is that many times my mother would say, "Well, I just got my period for the last time." She said that multiple times and it became this running joke for me, so much so that even my husband, Rodd, refers to it from time to time. He also remembers that each time she said it, it ended up not actually being the last time because she would say it again! I know that there were a few times she had gone more than twelve months between periods. That means, technically, that she was in menopause but still having occasional periods.

During the time she was likely menopausal, my mother got divorced for the second time. She was married to my father for twelve years and then to my stepfather for twenty years. She did share with me that she had really looked forward to having sex without any concern about becoming pregnant, but I never heard more about that after her second divorce. To my knowledge, she was never sexually active after that divorce, so she didn't have an opportunity to take advantage of menopausal contraception.

I am now fifty-four years old. I had an IUD placed for the first time five years ago, and I haven't had a period since the first few months after it was placed. Other than one year in my early twenties when I took the pill, I haven't taken any hormones and haven't used any hormonal birth control. I'll add here that I've been pregnant five times, and I have four children. I had a child who was stillborn, who would have been fourteen years old this year. Motherhood, intentional fertility, and avoiding hormones that would disrupt any natural process related to menstruation, pregnancy, and breastfeeding, have all been an important part of my identity.

I love that we are collaborating as menopause sisters where you have no children by choice, took the birth control pill for a few decades, and you've had noteworthy symptoms that definitely got your attention while I have four children, only took the pill briefly, and really haven't had any symptoms.

To be more precise, I thought I had no symptoms and really didn't think of myself as menopausal until the two of us started talking. I didn't think of myself as non-menopausal, either. I just didn't have any attention on it. But now, because we're talking about menopause, I realize I am definitely menopausal, and I have a very small collection of symptoms that may be related to menopause.

Tricia: Oh?

Alexandra: Beginning three years ago, I became dizzy on a few different occasions. Once I was on the highway, I needed to pull over. It was very scary. Probably because I'm a physician, I found myself considering my symptoms at the same time I was having them. I wondered if I was having a stroke. But I wasn't, and my dizziness just passed.

This happened two or three more times while I was coaching on Zoom. One time I remember coaching a couple and having to put my head down. It felt rather unprofessional in the moment, but I just had to do it. Since it wasn't a stroke the first time, I thought it might be the beginning of menopause. But it only happened a handful of times, and I forgot about it until recently.

In our ears, we have estrogen receptors, which is an explanation for why vertigo is particularly common during menopause. But when it didn't happen again, and nothing else happened, I considered it a quirky thing and didn't put any further attention on it until now.

In the last year, I've also noticed sweating a lot at night. It's not the kind of night sweats that wake me up; there's no drenching the sheets or needing to change my nightgown. It's more that I feel sweatier than I ever used to when I wake up. It's not specifically unpleasant, but it wasn't pleasant either, so I started paying attention to possible causes.

I noticed it was associated with my eating a lot of carbohydrates the day before. Recently I've largely been avoiding bread and grain-related products. But when I do eat them, I definitely notice that I sweat more during the night. However, a few days ago, I looked it up. It turns out that carbohydrates enhance menopause symptoms, and one of the ways to minimize menopause symptoms is going on a keto or paleo diet or something similar. So even though I haven't thought of my occasional increase in sweating at night as a symptom of menopause, it could well be.

Tricia: Wow, I've never heard about the connection between carbohydrates and menopause before. I find it quite interesting.

Alexandra: I think so too.

I'm also pretty sure I have what would qualify as brain fog. But again, I didn't initially recognize it as a symptom of menopause.

I used to take for granted having an outstanding memory. I'll give you an example. I once did a training that involved meeting in person for one weekend a month for ten months. There were 150 people in the training with me. During the second weekend, I was looking down while taking notes when the woman teaching said, "Who here knows every single person's name?" I put my hand up without looking up because I was still taking notes on what had been said before. With my head down, I had assumed that at least half the people there would have raised their hands, but when I looked up, I saw that no one had—not even one other person had raised their hand.

The presenter said, "Okay, come up here." When I got to the front of the room, she handed me the mic and told me to say each person's name. I turned to face the audience and went one by one, just missing one person and otherwise correctly stating each person's name.

Tricia: 150 names? Oh my God.

Alexandra: Yes. I am telling you this because that was my normal. I didn't think anything of it. I used to take very few notes when I would coach because I always remembered what I'd told people and what people had told me. But lately, in the last year or so, I've noticed that occasionally I'll tell a story and won't have remembered having shared it before. It doesn't happen with things other people tell me as much as it does with what I have shared with someone else. Also, I definitely don't remember people's names as well, or as quickly, anymore.

I said something about this to my husband, Rodd, telling him I was a bit concerned about losing my memory. It's not that I think I have early-onset dementia or anything like that, but I have definitely seen a decline. Rodd's response is that my memory used to be extraordinary, and now it's more like most people's!

Tricia: Do you think it's related to menopause specifically or just the natural aging process?

Alexandra: I have a coach who has an incredibly high level of attention and the kind of memory I used to have. I've been working with her for about a year and a half. She always remembers what I've told her. One day I started to say something, and she said, "Oh, yes, you told me about that earlier." Initially, it really surprised me and threw me for a loop. But now I am used to it as it's become my usual.

Initially, when this kind of thing would happen, I thought it was the result of my life being so wonderfully full that there was just too much to retain everything. So I didn't attribute it to either menopause or the natural aging process.

I remember being in sixth grade and having a substitute teacher who talked about the mind being like a bureau. As you learn things and have experiences, you put things in the drawers. Once the drawers are full, things start falling out the back of the bureau, and you just keep putting things in. But the bureau can't expand. You can stuff things in and squeeze things into back corners, but inevitably, there are going to be socks and underwear and shirts falling out the back of the bureau because it can only hold so much. This was her metaphor for memory, and it came into my consciousness after about forty years and gave me a way to relate to what was happening to me.

Tricia: Maybe she was in menopause?

Alexandra: Ha, ha, maybe! That's fun to consider because it most definitely wasn't in my mind when I first heard this!

It's probably something I remembered all those years ago precisely because it was so different from my own experience. I couldn't imagine being exposed to new knowledge and not being able to fit it all into my mind. The concept was comical and foreign to me. However, it was my main reference point when this started to happen to me. So I concluded, well, my life is so full of fascination and nuance, and intricacy with human beings, and my internal world is full of reflections and insight–it must be too much to fit in the "bureau" of my mind.

I really do have a very full life with my attention on many different landscapes. There's my husband and our four children, two of whom don't live at home. I'm aware of each of their lives in terms of what is happening and also what they are internally chewing on at any given moment. As a veteran homeschooler, I'm also tracking what my homeschooled children are learning as I have an eye on their day-to-day lessons, as well as their overall academic progress. I am also deeply immersed in the worlds of each of my clients. I am aware of their children and the dynamics in their relationships, and all the various narratives that are relevant as I coach them. So at any given time, I have my attention on a lot of different worlds within me. Understandably, I thought my bureau might have become too full to retain everything.

After becoming aware of this trend, I decided to multitask less and focus my attention more deeply on one thing at a time in order to see if that made a difference. It's a little bit helpful but hasn't really changed my overall situation.

Another thing I've noticed has to do with word retrieval. I've always been extremely articulate and enjoyed a rather varied and expansive vocabulary. Now, sometimes, I can't think of a word. Once again, I never associated this with menopause until we started working on this book. I thought of it as some combination of having a really rich life, and aging, although those two are related because the cumulative effect of a rich life is that there's going to be more and more in the bureau. That sums up how I thought about this until you and I started talking about menopause and its impact.

Tricia: And then?

Alexandra: Then I started thinking, for the very first time, "Oh, maybe these are menopausal symptoms." But I think it doesn't actually matter that much except for two reasons. One is that if it is menopause, then perhaps my memory will grow stronger again once my hormones find their new postmenopausal normal. The other way in which it matters is that I find attributing these changes to menopause has me feeling a deeper kinship with other women. I wasn't missing that kinship, even as I enjoy noticing I have it when I think about it in this way.

Tricia: I love the distinction you've made, Alexandra, between seeing menopause as pathological versus menopause as just a moment in time. I think that's really important. As you talk about it, it makes me think that I've never identified moments where I can't think of someone's name as potentially connected to menopause. So perhaps they are, but I want to know from you, how does that feel? And how are you taking care of yourself in the context of this change?

Alexandra: Well, when it first began, I'd kind of slap myself (in a way that was imperceptible to anyone else). I was disgusted because a piece of my identity was wrapped up in being aware of people and their stories and being able to remember names and other details. I had tied together my ability to put attention on someone and remember who they are and what they said with how I expressed my care for people.

Not being able to do that anymore, I did have some self-loathing. In not remembering people's names and forgetting whether I had already said something to someone, I became cognizant of new behaviors in me. They felt insensitive and disconnected. Self-loathing is perhaps too strong. It was more that I watched myself while being disgusted. Honestly, that was a relatively short phase, as I fairly quickly transitioned into thinking of it as something I need to accommodate. In other words, I became matter-of-fact about it.

Now, I give myself grace and compensate as elegantly as possible by casually and carefully beginning a story with "I'm not sure if I've told you this before. If I have, please interrupt me."

Tricia: Got it. I want to focus more on this being a concern you had.

Alexandra: Well, my mother was fifty-five when she first discovered a lump in her breast. While there were many phases, and she lived another five years, that was essentially the beginning of the end. It's quite significant for me because I'm now fifty-four. For about twenty years, I've been anticipating this time in my life, partly dreading it and partly feeling hopeful that I could have an experience different from my mother's.

I have made a point of engaging in positive self-talk and have prioritized a healthy mindset and healthy habits as much as I am able. To get to the point, I would say that the fact my mother died at sixty, after basically being sick the majority of her time from age fifty-five to age sixty, has left me feeling that being healthy now is a big win and definitely not to be taken for granted!

Tricia: Absolutely. And I'm wondering if our self-care practices, including affirming self-talk, along with our overall positive outlook, are why we are having the kind of menopause experiences we're having.

My own mother had a terrible time. I just plain refused to step into those shoes. She really struggled. She was crying all the time and really emotional. I remember watching her go through all this and being completely intolerant. I didn't know what it was or how to manage my own feelings around it; it appeared indulgent, and that's on me because her experience was very real. It was her truth.

I wasn't able to support her in her truth. Regardless of my judgments, she needed to treat herself the way she decided to, in terms of listening to doctors, taking hormones, or anything else she did. I was clear that I was not going to go through menopause the way my mother had. In fact, I did go on to make my own decisions without being influenced by her.

I choose to adopt a very positive outlook in my personal life, generally, and that is especially true when it comes to menopause.

Alexandra: I did some incredible family constellation work around this. Have you heard of Bert Hellinger and his Family Constellations work?

Tricia: Yes, that's such powerful work.

Alexandra: It's incredibly powerful work.

Some years after my mother died, I did a session because I realized that I was walking around, waiting until it was my turn to get breast cancer. As I mentioned, my mother died from breast cancer. My maternal grandmother also died from breast cancer. With this lineage, I found myself believing that I was living my life while waiting for it to be my turn. One day I achieved enough objectivity to realize that was ridiculous.

I arranged to participate in a family constellation session with someone who specializes in working with medical issues. My goal was to shed the sense of inevitability that I would be diagnosed with breast cancer and die from it. The session was very efficient and totally profound. The way Family Constellation therapy works is you basically use the other people present to create a vignette with the characters from your family. In the therapeutic vignette, you get to rewrite the script and create a new outcome.

I chose a woman who was there to represent my mother and a man to represent my husband. The woman representing my mother stood in front of me, and the man representing my husband sat beside me. I began by facing forward, locking eyes with the woman representing my mother. I had my full attention on her, feeling my love for my mother and expressing my loyalty to her through my undivided attention.

The transformational, therapeutic moment came as I consciously turned my gaze away from my mother and intentionally turned toward my husband. It might seem very simple to transfer my attention, but making that shift was one of the hardest things I have ever done. It represented a kind of disconnecting from my beloved mother and turning the majority of my attention to the present and the future. I brought myself to Rodd, who also represented our family and our life together. The Family Constellations therapist set it up artfully; this act of turning towards my husband, and all it meant, was pivotal beyond measure. It was definitive.

Now, instead of feeling like my days are numbered and I'm just waiting for my breast cancer diagnosis, I have an attitude of "Sure, I might get breast cancer, but I am not just waiting for it, and life is wonderfully full right now."

Tricia: Wow, what a shift.

Alexandra: It truly was.

This makes me think of a quote I love from Brianna Wiest: "True self-care is not salt baths and chocolate cake. It is making the choice to build a life you don't need to regularly escape from."

That quote is so relevant to this conversation. I've noticed that many women live while putting aside things that are important to them. They hold off on partaking in longed-for experiences, going for their dreams, and making decisions that foster self-respect. Then, seemingly all of a sudden, during menopause, there is a second chance to pursue these things. With the emergence of a new identity, finally, and maybe for the first time, a woman chooses to prioritize herself. She feels it's time to wake up because if not then, when?

Tricia: I think menopause presents a moment of deep reflection. I'm wondering, when you think about moving into that reflection, and you think about having had children, what do you think about now? How do you relate to the reality that it is no longer an option for you and Rodd to have any more biological children? Have you thought about it? Have you created a ceremony to honor the transition? As a mother of four, what does this look and feel like for you?

Alexandra: It's a great question, and it hasn't really been an issue one way or the other.

When we had our first child, Josephine, I knew immediately that we would have another child. Christopher was born two years later. At the time, we were both working many hours, about seventy to one hundred hours a week. With those schedules, it just didn't make sense to have more children, so we decided that Rodd would get a vasectomy.

A few years later, when we were done with medical training and our work schedules were more civilized, we wanted more children, and Rodd had a vasectomy reversal. Within the year, Gabriel was born. A few years later, we conceived Jacob. He was stillborn, and I almost died while giving birth to him.

It took a long time to heal from that experience, physically and emotionally, but eventually, we were back on track with my health, our intimacy and sex, and other elements we really cared about in our relationship. While I still didn't feel our family was complete, we decided not to have any more children in order to keep going with the forward momentum of our marriage.

A few years later, I went to a retreat. In a guided visualization about our deepest desires, I found myself flooded with the truth of my desire to have another child. When I returned home, I told Rodd, saying, "I think we're meant to have another baby." He is amazing and said, "Okay, well, let's give it a try." We were both forty-three years old, and that night, Matthew was conceived.

I share all of this to provide meaningful context when I say that when he was born, I felt something new. I felt totally clear in my knowing that our family was complete; it was very joyful for me. I didn't know I was ever going to have that feeling, but I did. I still do.

So, no, I don't ever wish I could have another baby. I do love giving birth. I love being pregnant. But no part of me has any desire to raise more children. This means there really is no loss for me in menopause in that regard.

After his vasectomy reversal, Rodd and I agreed that he wouldn't have another procedure on his genitals. Instead, after our youngest child was born, I had an IUD placed. I was ready to have it removed recently, but my doctor said, "Why

don't you leave it in for another year?" While I am not likely
to menstruate, there was a chance that I might have periods
once the IUD was removed. If there was a chance I might,
she thought I might as well just leave the IUD in and thereby
experience a simpler, more straightforward menopause.

She's a doctor. I'm a doctor. We both knew it could come out,
and I'd have no symptoms. Or it could come out, and I might
have a lot of bleeding. I haven't had my hormones checked
and don't actually know what they are. However, since I feel
fine, I thought I might as well leave the IUD in me for another
two years. That way, when it is finally removed, I expect I'll be
on the other side of menopause.

The truth is, menopause symptoms can be non-existent.
They can also go on for a few months or years. It's not that
unusual for a woman to experience seven years of hot flashes.
The average age of menopause is fifty-one, but some women
menstruate into their sixties. The point is, when it comes to
menopause, normal can look many different ways.

Tricia: So much range.

Alexandra: Yes. Truly.

I'll add that our oldest child is twenty-six years old, and our
youngest child is eleven. We definitely look forward to being
empty nesters and entering that next phase of life. However,
I can remember about eleven or twelve years ago, Rodd asked
what I thought would hold us together once our children were
out of the house. At the time, our lives were so interwoven with

our children's—these were the years of having a baby in diapers, a child under the age of seven, and years of homeschooling teenagers. It was all a huge energetic investment, and I gave it my all. I remember when Rodd asked that, I was kind of shocked because I thought for sure we would have an amazing life together once our children grew up. It wasn't a question I had at all. But when he said that, it got me thinking.

In many ways, his question was the beginning of a growing commitment to tend our marriage more than ever before in incredibly beautiful ways. Our sex and intimacy, our conversations, and the amount of fun we have together have all greatly improved.

I'm reminded of a confronting statistic, namely, that the average couple spends less than four minutes a day talking about anything other than children and logistics. I think we were better than many couples in that regard, but even so, his wondering about the future was a huge wake-up call for me. It wasn't a dramatic wake-up call. It wasn't painful. I was just very glad to see what was happening in his mind because it was very different from what was happening in my mind.

Now, after having used his question as a springboard to really improve the foundation of our relationship, we've expanded our shared identities well beyond being parents. When we talk about how it will be when it's just the two of us, when all the children are out of the house, Rodd gets a big grin on his face. We love our children devotedly, and we also look forward to that time when they are all launched, and it's just the two of us again.

Tricia: That is so beautiful and powerful. It's lovely to hear that you feel so complete as a mother. And also that you can fully step into this new place as a fully realized mother and wife who is in menopause now.

Alexandra: You know, Tricia, I don't necessarily carry the identity of being in menopause.

Tricia: Really?

Alexandra: I think it's because it just hasn't meant that much to me one way or the other, and it hasn't come up in any conversation before you and I started speaking.

Ever since I was young, I have looked forward to being old. I've always been fascinated with getting older and wondered how it would be for me. I remember thinking when I was much younger, "Who am I going to be when I'm thirty?" "Who am I going to be when I'm forty?" "Who am I going to be when I'm fifty?" "How will I change?" "What will I think about?" "How will I live?" I looked forward to all of it with excitement and anticipation, never fear or dread.

I think what I'm saying is that menopause didn't really seem so interesting to me per se as compared to the general fascination I've felt about becoming older.

Another thing that plays into this has to do with appearances. When I was around the age of sixteen, I realized that most of the women I knew spent a certain, relatively short portion of their life wanting to look and appear older than they were. Thereafter they wanted to appear younger than they were. I observed that and found it absurd. Since making that observation, I have never tried to look younger or older than my actual biological age.

This is all to say that I don't resist being in menopause. But I hadn't really given it much attention before you invited me into this collaboration to write a book on the topic. In many ways, I see that menopause has been unacknowledged by me, although there hasn't been anything definitive that's changed since I haven't had a period in about five years. I wonder if this lack of attention to menopause is the case for many women.

Tricia: Oh, that makes sense. And I love that your experience is so different from my own.

Alexandra: After this conversation, I expect I will identify as a woman in menopause. But at the moment, it still feels like a mantle I need to put on. Is it a mantle I want? I'm not sure. I may have some unconscious resistance at play, which I will definitely investigate.

In my life, I am often amazed, filled with awe and wonder, and enthusiasm for humanity in its many forms. However, I have associations with menopause as a state of being that is dry and dehydrated. Maybe that's the impact of societal conditioning

In any case, I definitely don't identify as a dehydrated woman, and I never want to. I want to remain open to being juicy, believing it is possible for the rest of my life.

Put more succinctly, to answer your question from a while back, yes, I am complete with my fertility. I am a yes to moving into the next phase of my life. For the first time in my life, I also feel quite powerful in my professional life. I see the significant, positive impact my contribution makes for couples through my work as a Relationship and Intimacy Coach and an Intimate Marriage Expert.

More than looking at menopause as an identity I might adopt, I have been thinking a lot about what bullshit we've all been fed about aging because the truth is that being in my fifties has been incredible so far!

chapter 4

HIDING IN PLAIN SIGHT

Alexandra: The medical definition of menopause, literally, is that there is no menstruation for twelve months. That is all there is to it. I'm realizing that the medical definition is flat, and I find myself wanting to talk more about the richness available in menopause. You have been talking about your thrill around it and sharing how you take what other people see as problematic symptoms and reframe them as enjoyable, or at least interesting, experiences.

Tricia: Yes, that's right. I started having night sweats when I was thirty-eight. I remember being in bed with my husband, Joe, and waking up completely drenched as if I had taken a shower. There were no warning signs, no preamble. This just suddenly happened.

Alexandra: Like a mature woman's wet dream?

Tricia: Not quite. Definitely not. Although I do remember one conversation early on, when I was drenched, and Joe said, "Honey, it's just hot in here. It's just the comforter." I remember thinking, "I'm gonna punch you right in the throat. It is NOT just the comforter. How dare you challenge my experience of my body at this moment?"

This thought lasted for less than thirty seconds because, once I explained what was going on, he adapted instantaneously. He became very used to me having night sweats. It got to the point where I would wake up drenched, and he would notice, get up, and bring me one of his t-shirts. Then I would sit up, put my arms up like a little kid, and he would strip off my wet shirt and put his dry shirt on me. Then I would go back to bed, and he would put a new blanket on me too. That was my experience with my amazing husband, especially once he understood, which hardly took much time. He loved me during this new phase of our relationship. Unconditionally.

Alexandra: Let's just pause for a moment.

This right here is one of the reasons this book is important for men to read. The issues are multi-dimensional and broadly relevant. The way your little girl energy got to participate in this very grown-up experience is gorgeous. You've invited all parts of you to go through the process with you. Both your inner child and your adult body got to participate.

I want to also highlight that it's not that Joe was enlightened in advance. It's that you chose to educate him with respect and kindness and no derision. Once he understood, your spectacular man got involved and participated in creating comfort for you. That is very, very important.

To make that point more clear, let's go back to before that was the case. You said you wanted to punch him in the throat? Can you give me a sense of what was going on inside you?

Tricia: That sounds so violent, and it's not actually what I wanted to do, but it does convey my frustration.

Joe is a very good learner. He is a quick study; it doesn't take a lot for him to understand something. I'm guessing it was probably the second or third time I said that I wasn't sweating because I was hot or the room was hot but rather because I was having a physiological experience. Once that became clear, he was completely on board and has been ever since.

Alexandra: He wasn't worried?

Tricia: No, he wasn't worried. He was solution driven.

It goes back to how we have approached all of these physiological changes. He didn't get up and go to the couch because it was wet in the bed. That would have made it seem that I was the problem, and I would have felt ashamed. It's not how we handled things. Joe was solution driven. He was loving and accepting. We both felt we were having the experience together.

Alexandra: It's really important to emphasize that your symptoms didn't become a source of disconnection. Much of what causes disconnection in relationships can actually be used to create more connection and more tenderness. This is such a great example of that.

Tricia: I have never thought about it this way. But really, it connected us more intimately; it felt good to allow him to take care of me. I let him in.

Alexandra: Yes, yes, yes you did. So sweetly too.

Tricia: That was new.

I am pretty much all masculine. I'm definitely an Alpha. When we moved into this apartment, I very consciously set things up in a way that would support me in accessing more feminine energy. Giving myself permission to be that feminine with him has served our relationship tremendously.

Alexandra: Part of an ambitious woman becoming more open to her man involves her willingness to give up control and allow herself to be taken care of, which is exactly what I'm hearing from you. You didn't wake up cursing. You didn't suddenly start hating your body. You didn't resent it. You went with it and allowed your husband to change your shirt.

Tricia: I did go with it, and I still go with it. It's been an incredible opportunity to witness who I am.

My progression from when I was thirty-eight to now has included consistent night sweats throughout. They have been cyclical, occurring probably every three months. It's been consistent and ongoing.

I've also had hot flashes, which are quite different from night sweats.

Alexandra: In what ways?

Tricia: With night sweats, you wake up drenched as if you've just run a marathon or taken a shower. With hot flashes, I can feel the heat being generated in my body, starting from my root chakra and rising to come out through my face, sometimes my armpits. It's very powerful and very sexy. It's like a life force moving through me.

Alexandra: Before an audition someone can feel nervous and nauseous, but in another circumstance, the exact same physical sensations can be interpreted as excitement and anticipation. Is it like that, where some people are super uncomfortable, and you're finding it sexy?

Tricia: Yes, it's like butterflies, which can be interpreted in a variety of ways. Great distinction.

Since we've brought Joe into this, it's making me think about something. He has a sweater that he wears when we're in the living room together because I often have the air conditioning on. He is so lovely about it. Sometimes he just says, "I'll be right back, honey, I'm gonna get my sweater." He does not say, "Why on earth is the air conditioning on again?" It's such a beautiful "we're in this together" gesture. He's so aligned that he's even written a line about this into the play he's writing.

Alexandra: Really? I love this.

Tricia: Yes, he's having a reading of it next week. It's about a family. The father, the patriarch, has lost his wife. After a year, he decides to sell the family home. He's sitting at the kitchen table, talking to his wife, who has transitioned, and he says, "Honey, I miss you so much. You always ran fifteen degrees hotter than me. I love when I used to reach over just to make sure that you were in bed next to me." The monologue feels like a special tribute to our relationship.

How we are together is so beautiful. To have that kind of love, joy, acceptance, and togetherness on this journey is beyond description. Joe's involvement in my menopausal evolution has contributed to my feelings of empowerment. I feel seen and held.

I'm not experiencing brain fog. I'm not experiencing sleeplessness. I'm not experiencing many of the things that many women experience in menopause. I honor the experiences of all women, but at the same time, I don't want to diminish my own experience and pretend it's not as great as it is. After all, it's my experience, it's perfectly valid, and I am definitely having a really good time. Menopausal experiences are individual and varied, and any woman's experience is true.

Alexandra: Yes.

Tricia: I'm curious to see what happens when I'm in a studio, rehearsing a show. With the pandemic, we haven't been doing that for the last two years, so I haven't experienced having a hot flash in front of other people.

I think about when my eyesight changed. I'd be sure to have a pair of reading glasses on hand so I could read the script. Then I would put them on the top of my head so I could look up and see the cast. I would make those adjustments matter of factly. I never apologized about it or ever thought of doing so. In fact, I enjoyed all the opportunities to wear sexy reading glasses. I really got into it. So when I think about going back into the studio to rehearse with speakers or actors, I picture treating it similarly. If I have, say, an explosion of upper lip sweat, I'll do a little dab, continue talking, and keep moving forward. Hot flashes are not going to prevent me from being creative or being at the helm of the ship. I feel no need to hide it.

Alexandra: Normalizing is empowering.

Tricia: Absolutely.

Alexandra: This reminds me of something I often talk about. My father was a single man living in Manhattan for seven years before he married my mother. Four years later, I was born. At the time, my father felt certain he had never seen a single stroller in all his years living in Manhattan. But once he had me in a stroller, he saw strollers everywhere, on every street. There were suddenly so many strollers! I feel similarly about menopause. It's not something I was aware of. It's not something I perceived in my interactions with people. Sometimes, even women going through it aren't really seeing it. But it's been here all along! It's hiding in plain sight and present everywhere.

Tricia: I love that. Yes, it's hiding in plain sight.

chapter 5

MENOPAUSE IN THE WORKPLACE

A CONVERSATION WITH PAT DUCKWORTH

Tricia: We're super honored and excited to be able to have this conversation with you, Pat, so thank you so much for joining us.

Pat: It's really good to be here.

Alexandra: Welcome.

Tricia: First, would you start by sharing a little about yourself? We've done our research, but we would love to hear you tell your story too. Please tell us how you got into this field and the kinds of situations you work with.

Pat: I'm Pat Duckworth. I'm based here in the UK, just south of Cambridge. I'm a women's wellness and workplace menopause specialist. I've been working in this area for about ten years. I've written five books on the subject of menopause. Prior to getting into this field, I worked in public service for over thirty years. When I got to menopause, I realized I wanted to do something different. I wanted to retrain in another field.

When you find yourself crying on the way to work, you know something is horribly wrong. One day I came home and told my husband, "I need to do something very different." He responded, "Great, what are you going to do?"

I'd always been interested in neurolinguistic programming, so I committed to a ten-month course that met one weekend a month. When I had a chance to take early retirement, I leaped at the opportunity. So by the time I'd finished my training, I was ready to start a new business. I became a therapist and coach, then decided I wanted to write a book. I thought to myself, "What do I know a lot about?" At that time, I knew a lot about menopause.

My first book for women was titled *Hot Women, Cool Solutions*. It's about how to use mind-body techniques to help get through menopause. Back then, from 2010 to 2012, the conversation around menopause was pretty sparse. As I grew my business, I would go to networking meetings and say, "I help women in menopause." The response was like a tumbleweed rolling across the room. People would ask, "Why would you do that? What? What on earth is that about?"

I gave my first talk on menopause in the workplace in 2015 to a big government department. At the time, there was one piece of workplace menopause research. Now, seven years later, the conversation in the UK is so strong around workplace menopause, and menopause in general, that you can hardly move without tripping over another piece of research concerning menopause and the effects it has in the workplace. In the ten years I've been working in this area, the landscape has changed enormously.

Tricia: This is fascinating for me because I've never worked for anyone else, and I've never even considered this would be a conversation that wasn't happening.

Pat: I hear that from entrepreneurs quite frequently. They also sometimes wonder what there is to say about it, but the topic actually arises quite organically.

I've worked with all sorts of organizations, from firefighters to government departments to commercial housebuilders. If department heads were employing a lot of women, they started to think, "Hmm, are we losing women at this stage of life? Are we getting the same bang for our buck? Are we missing a trick here?" There is so much evidence available now which proves that if you support women at this stage of life, you can retain really knowledgeable, experienced women for many more years. You also have a happier workforce, and the whole atmosphere improves for everyone, including all the men who work with women.

Alexandra: Would you give an example of how this plays out? Let's say there's a male CEO of a company with ten employees and another one with 30,000 employees. What would happen in each of these companies that would trigger these male CEOs, or for that matter female CEOs, to look into the resources that are available? What is the observation that triggers someone to reach out to you (as opposed to you being on a panel or someone reading one of your books and therefore happening to learn about menopause in the workplace)?

Pat: One of the big organizations I've worked with is the Cheshire Fire and Rescue Service. I don't know how many people it employs, but it is a big fire service in the UK. Their Chief Fire Officer was very engaged with equality, diversity, and inclusion. He looked around at his workforce and wondered, "How can we make this more diverse and inclusive?"

This led him to set up a women's support group. From that women's support group came new questions and considerations. What could they do with even more support around women's hormonal health? If you've got women who are firefighters, and they're out on site, what do they need that is different from what men need? How do we retain the women that are in the back offices?

In this particular company, the Chief Fire Officer had a male firefighter whose female partner was having a really difficult time in menopause. It was affecting the male firefighter's performance in the workplace. Firefighters work in shifts, and if this firefighter isn't getting sleep because he's taking his wife to various appointments and he's worried about her job too, then he's not going to perform as well as he otherwise would.

An example of a smaller company I consulted with had a different situation. The CEO's wife was having a lot of trouble with her menopause. He started asking around, which is unusual for a male CEO, but he was concerned, and he wanted to understand what was going on. He talked to his head of Human Resources and told her they should be thinking about menopause in terms of their workforce.

An even smaller company, one with only half a dozen people, was run by a woman. We really shouldn't assume that women are more tuned in to this than men are because, honestly, you can have as many problems with a female manager or business owner as you would with a male manager. It makes no difference. But in this instance, one of her key employees was having trouble. She was very young, and she'd gone into early menopause. This employee was having trouble concentrating. She was making mistakes. She was sweating in meetings. She was experiencing a whole bunch of symptoms. The manager started to really engage with her about what was going on because the employee was a key member of the team, and the manager wanted her to be working well.

Alexandra: I have a very uninformed question.

Pat: Go for it.

Alexandra: I'm a physician. I hear what you're saying. And I think, well, it sounds like people need quality medical care. There is definitely a real problem with doctors not being educated about menopause. So I'm not saying it's an easy fix for people to get good care, but you're in the UK, where everyone has insurance and access to doctors. Given that, I am over here thinking, well, the government really needs to provide proper education for doctors. That's the way to handle this because menopause is a medical issue. But you're not saying that at all. You're saying something quite different.

I want to say something like, "Pretend I'm five years old and explain how you think about this, with menopause not being an individual medical issue but rather a systemic work environment issue." I'd love to make the leap and see it through your eyes.

Pat: To begin with, there is another piece of the puzzle to understand. Here in the UK, we have the Equality Act of 2010. The Equality Act is about making sure that employers treat people equally. There are a number of "protected characteristics." In other words, you can't discriminate against people in the workplace on the basis of any of these characteristics. Age is a characteristic, gender is a characteristic, and disability is a characteristic. If you take those three together, you run straight into menopause.

Although menopause isn't a disability per se, some employees have called out their employers and even taken legal action saying, "I was discriminated against on the basis of my menopause." Such discrimination is covered by the act based on age and gender. In my own experience, even though I was getting medical treatment, I was unable to function because my symptoms were so bad. It was a disability, accommodations weren't made, and therefore I was discriminated against. You have to keep all that in the back of your mind.

Honestly, for some employers, the motivation is wanting to avoid any legal action taken against them. But that motivation only became relevant once women began bringing these issues to the fore, which led to multiple successful court cases. Some women have been campaigning on this, and advocating for everyone, as it's become part of our legislation; it's written into our code of law.

Employers are required to consider reasonable adjustments if somebody has a problem in the workplace or a disability. What can employers reasonably do to help them? With menopause, this has led to consulting with employees about what would help them. The answers are individual because not everybody wants to have a fan on their desk. Some people do because they have hot flashes, but not necessarily every woman of a certain age.

Imagine it—you're sitting in an office, you're in your late forties, and you've worked for that employer for approximately twenty years. You're a valued member of the team. In this context, you might say, "If I could just have a fan on my desk, I'd feel better." The employer is going to respond by putting a fan on your desk.

Or take being able to go to the bathroom when you want. Not every employer is as accommodating as they could be. If you're working in retail, you might be told there are specific times you can have breaks. But if you're experiencing heavy bleeding because of your menopause or your bladder is not as strong as it used to be, you might not last until the next break.

In that situation, a reasonable adjustment would be that you can go to the bathroom when you want to.

Another reasonable adjustment is having access to cold drinking water when you need it. Or if you wear a uniform, it might be that you need to change from one made of polyester to one made of cotton with better aeration. Maybe you have a shirt that's up to your ears, with cuffs past your wrists, and you are sweating–you're going to need something different to wear. These kinds of reasonable workplace adjustments are important. I hope you can see this isn't just a medical issue.

Alexandra: You are a magnificent spokesperson for this consideration. I have learned so much from your answer.

Pat: Thank you.

In the last couple of years, particularly during lockdown, when employers were trying to retain their employees, we've seen that companies are becoming much more constructive and creative. For example, an employer might be offering yoga classes during lunch breaks because they know it's good for the women in the organization. Men can go as well, but it's mostly women going because the classes provide somewhere women can lie down in the middle of the day when they are experiencing cliff edge fatigue. They need to lie down, or they are going to collapse over their desks. Lunchtime yoga classes are an elegant accommodation.

Here in England, you still have to pay a prescription charge to take hormone therapy. Some employers have said, "We think this is so important that we're going to pay your prescription charge. If you need to go to the doctor or a medical consultant, you can have time off to do that."

Something else women find quite helpful is flexible working hours. They want to work the same number of hours, but if they could come in earlier, when they feel a bit brighter, and go home a bit earlier, it would make a huge difference. For other women, they just want to stay in bed an extra hour because they're so tired. They can go to work later in the afternoon and miss rush hour on the way back. Flexible working hours are a real bonus for a lot of women.

Tricia: Wow, every one of these considerations sounds so obvious.

It seems you've been able to communicate this quite effectively to so many organizations, such that now they fully incorporate these adjustments. How long did it take for you to do that?

Pat: Well, it's been ten years since I started working in this field. In 2015, I gave my first talk about it. The central government, local government, some of the armed services, firefighters, and ambulance corps were early adopters, partly because trade unions were involved. At the same time, other movements were growing that led to encouraging people to speak up about workplace menopause support, with more advocates for it. However, I have to say that legal cases decided in favor of women, and women receiving compensation, really made a difference. Lawsuits can be damaging to a brand, and these cases cause companies to act quickly.

In reality, most of the cases have resulted in very small settlement amounts compared to the size of the business. But the damage to the brand is far more costly. "How have you treated your women?" is a question they want to answer well. Plus, most of the lawsuits have gone to court. You read them, and you wonder how the manager didn't know this was a problem. How did they not get it? It seems so obvious when you read the case.

We have had some pushback too. It's from men, and some women too. It always disappoints me when it's from leading women who say, "These women who take these cases to court just make things worse for the rest of us." I say, no, they're not. They are trying to break through barriers.

There was a case last year where a woman was working for a small company. She was in her late forties or early fifties. It was a small family business, but she wasn't one of the family. The owner, a man, disrespected her. With customers present, he would shout from his office, saying, "Oh, this is all about your menopause." "These menopausal women…". I think he did it a couple of times. The employee went to his wife, who also worked in the business. She said, "This is unacceptable. I don't want him saying this kind of thing. It's ridiculous." The wife responded along the lines of "Just suck it up." Can you believe it? This woman was awarded compensation and damages.

That was just a small company. But some of the lawsuits have involved pretty big companies. In one case, with a very big American company, a woman was passed over for promotion. She was very experienced, but the promotion went to somebody younger. I think male as well. Anyway, she asked to see her employment records and saw that it said she was a low-flight risk. In other words, because she was an older woman, she was going nowhere. Therefore they could pass her over for promotion. She, too, was awarded a lot of compensation because she was a more senior executive and more qualified, and the discrimination was clear.

Alexandra: Was that specifically a menopause matter?

Pat: Well, in that situation, it wasn't specifically. But I see it potentially being related because even though menopause wasn't mentioned, the kind of derogatory remarks around whether she would be likely to leave or not all pointed in that direction.

Tricia: Pat, the work you're doing is awesome!

There's been so much shame put on women about becoming older. How do you feel about the issue of shame and the notion that older women need to disappear or just suck it up if they want to participate in life?

Pat: That's all ageism. Women try to mask how old they are in order to avoid that, or in order to get the opportunities and respect that younger women are getting. Yet, strangely enough, we all get older every day. It's a good thing. I mean, it's a much better option than dying.

Tackling ageism in the workplace, particularly for women who have hit menopause, can be complicated because some very normal challenges can coexist. Women can begin to experience brain fog. They feel like they're getting dementia. They can't talk about it with anybody because they're embarrassed and afraid of what that could mean for their goals and livelihoods, for their lives. They're not going to say to their superiors or co-workers, "By the way, I got to the top of the stairs the other day, and I couldn't remember why I got there. I think I'm getting dementia." If they said that to a friend, the friend might say, "I get it. I do that every day. I couldn't even remember the kids' names yesterday."

There are so many aspects of menopause which are a completely normal part of aging, which can be really challenging, particularly if you're doing a senior executive job. No one wants to be seen as not functioning well. But if we talk about it, if we can get it out there, and communicate that this is what happens, we will get through it, and we'll be fine. We will get to the other side of it. If women knew this, if everyone knew this, we could remove some of the fear. Women who are simply getting older every day, as people do, do not have to view it as an embarrassment, concern, or emergency. Does that make sense?

Tricia: Do you feel that part of the changes that will help remove the fear around menopause must take place not only privately, at home, or in isolation, but in the workplace too?

Pat: Yes! There's absolutely no question. When I made my decision to jump ship from the public sector, where I had worked for decades, I could not have talked about my menopause with my boss. I just could not. I was a director in Her Majesty's Revenue and Customs, the equivalent of the IRS. I was experiencing brain fog. I wasn't having bad symptoms, so I wasn't rushing to a medical practitioner to get hormone therapy. I was actually very reluctant about that because my mother had breast cancer and she had had blood clotting. I'd already done my research and thought hormones were not for me. But I was getting brain fog. I felt like the world had gone out of focus. I felt I needed new glasses every day. Eventually, when I told my boss that my aunt had died, and I was her next of kin and executor, and I would need some time off, he said to me, "Oh, well, actually, a lot of it's online now. So it shouldn't be a problem for you." I thought, am I going to share my menopause with him? No way.

I don't want other women to be in that same position. I want women to be able to get support if they need support. I thought, what if the stigma wasn't there? What if it wasn't a taboo, and we could just say, "This is what I'm experiencing. And this is what would be helpful for me."

In recent years, there's been a lot of work done around mental health and mental health in the workplace. A lot of organizations in the UK have Mental Health First Aiders. If you're experiencing mental health problems, you can go and talk to them without any stigma. In workplaces, we now have menopause champions who are equivalent. It's not in every organization, but in some organizations, there is a person who serves as a contact point for women to talk to and be given resources. The menopause champion isn't sought out for medical issues; they are not there to give advice. Their function is to point people to resources and the relevant organizations that can help them. It's an amazing service.

Alexandra: That sounds exquisitely humane. You're thoughtful and articulate, and everything you share is really eye-opening. I'm excited and inspired!

As we have this opportunity to speak with you, I'd like to bring up another concern to hear how you respond. I have four children, and I'm sensitized to how birth, in our culture anyway, is seen as a medical diagnosis. When it comes to workplace policies and protocols, pregnancy and birth are viewed as illnesses. To state the obvious, I don't think of normal pregnancy and birth as illnesses, and I find it unfortunate that they are characterized as such by human resource departments. This view doesn't seem to be evolving in a way that honors the reality of women while also accounting for institutional needs. Seeing pregnancy as a pathology is an entrenched attitude that is reinforced in all kinds of ways and within multiple spheres.

I've shared that by way of providing context for my concern about the beautiful progress being made around menopause. You're showing a way forward that is fundamentally humane, but with it comes the inevitability that part of a woman's life is seen as a form of pathology that needs attention. How do you think about this consideration?

Pat: Menopause is a natural stage of life. We don't want to pathologize teenagers, right, or the process of going through puberty. Adolescence is not an illness. But some people experience it with quite a lot of challenges. That's where menopausal women are as well. They are going through normal changes but at another time in life. Sometimes it can be quite difficult.

If we really start educating teenagers and younger people about adolescence, it would be wonderful. We could say, "You're going through a natural stage of life. It feels horrible. You may have wanted it or not wanted it. Some kids would rather not become teenagers, and some can't wait. They want all of the exciting things that come with being more grown up. Some will get a few pimples, and others will have terrible acne. But, whatever it comes with, terrible or wonderful, exciting or horrifying, everyone has to go through it." That's how we need to look at menopause as well. Some of you might be welcoming it. You don't want periods anymore. You don't want to worry about getting pregnant. Others dread it. This is where I feel I am an ambassador because I am well on the other side of it and glad to share how glorious it is.

I'm having a brilliant life, having more fun than I think I ever did when I was younger. I'm traveling the world talking about this stuff. I'm glad to tell any woman, "I know this can feel horrible, but you will get to the other side." We have a generation of younger people who are more open to talking about all kinds of things anyway. The generation coming up behind me has had more support around pregnancy and fertility than earlier generations, been more open about their fertility issues, been more open about their pregnancies, their gender decisions, and all of that. Now they are coming into menopause, and they're bringing the same attitudes.

They ask. "What's going on here? What is this about? Why weren't we educated about this, and why isn't there an app?" I think the sort of technology that has gone with other parts of our reproductive life means these women are coming forward saying, "I want an app or other resources to deal with menopause too. I'm going to get to the other side of it, and I want to be informed. Not only that, but maybe I'll have forty or fifty years of living on the other side of it, so what have you got for me?"

Tricia: This is amazing. So amazing. How do you wrap your head around all of these women and their workplaces dismissing them or considering them damaged?

I know there's more to the work you're doing than providing allowances for menopausal symptoms. What else are you working on? What else are these workplace environments doing besides just allowing people to put fans on their desks? Is there something happening underneath, some bigger growth or change poking through?

Pat: Well, this is a dangerous time of life for women. Many of them get to the point I was wherein they are going through physical, mental, and spiritual changes all at the same time. When I talk about spiritual changes, people tend to mix that up with religion and wonder what a religious change could mean. I'm talking about something more like a transformational rite of passage that can shake you to your very foundation. Women may come out on the other side of menopause very committed to what they are doing now, or they may come out of the other side of it with something like, "You know what?

I've always wanted to be an eco-warrior. I'm going to do it! I don't care what anybody else thinks." That's the wonderful thing about getting to the other side of it. If it matters to you, you just go for it.

In the book I wrote last year, *Menopause: Mind the Gap*, I included a section on the necessity of coaching, or other ways of supporting women at this age, because women might begin to question their purpose. They may not be prepared for that. A lot of the identities we have around being a mother, a caretaker, a reproductive unit, a sex goddess—the identities that organize so much of the way we live and influence our live—they just fall away. Suddenly women are saying, "I don't know who I am anymore." Such identity shifts and questions can be quite intense. Really, it's an opportunity to say, but who do you want to be? What would be most fulfilling for you now?

This is challenging for women to find out. They wonder, "If all those identities are gone, everything that seemed to be really important has fallen away. Who am I now? Who do I want to be going forward for the next twenty, thirty, or forty years?" I think that is the other side of it, and it can be quite complicated.

So many of the words used for this stage of life, namely, "crone," "wise woman," and "senior," have been degraded. I mean, who wants to be a crone? Yet the derivation of the word is a person who's been crowned. In non-Western cultures, the women who are the grandmothers are revered for their knowledge and understanding. It's so important for some women to be introduced to that concept because they are so frightened that they are becoming invisible. They're not actually becoming invisible—it's just that all the old identities are falling away, and they don't know who they are anymore.

Alexandra: I'm appreciating that you shared enough context for our conversation to get here. Menopause as the journey of emerging identity is such a clear description. The way you've presented it is stunning. You have stimulated, inspired, and opened us up. While neither Tricia nor I are menopause experts beyond our respective experiences, we deeply resonate with this point.

Tricia: We do.

Pat: In large part, our purpose, values, beliefs, and capabilities develop our identities. Our brains organize themselves around those identities so that we are familiar with ourselves. If our basic identities feel like they are falling away, we lose that organization. We can feel incredibly out of sorts. Then we have to really tap into deeply important inquiries. We have to ask, "What is my purpose? What's the best version of me, and how can I begin to build that up now?" In many ways, that's the fun and adventure in all of this. It's where the juiciness is. We have to create the environment, the supportive environment, the culture within organizations, where that is possible. You can stimulate this from a lower level, but you need buy-in at the top. If you don't have buy-in from the top of an organization, you end up with pinkwashing.

Tricia: You're highlighting for me one of the reasons Alexandra and I are writing this book. We are each at the top of our fields. By speaking out and talking about our personal experiences in this way, we want to give other women permission to speak out as well.

Pat: That's where I was going—we have to role model how to navigate this. We have to role model it for other women. It's one of the reasons I don't sit in the corner, eat chocolate, and drink beer all the time. I want to show other women that you can discover your new identity and lead your life with joy.

When it comes to modeling for other women, that's not something I've just begun. Even when I was working my way through the ranks of public service, I never said, "Oh, look at me, I'm a woman." But all the while, I was role modeling. I was showing that you can get on quite well. I'd say, "I'm going to do this, I'm going to do that, I'm about to take these steps." Various women would watch me and later tell me, "You've been such a role model and inspiration for me." I never set out to do that. I just lived my life the way I wanted to, which is exactly what I'm doing now. I don't get up every morning thinking I'm a menopause warrior. I think, "I'm gonna live my life. If other people take inspiration from it, then I trust I've done a good job."

There's a Chief Fire Officer, one of only twenty fire officers in the UK. He loved going to meetings with members of parliament or senior colleagues. At one meeting, they were talking about firefighters working past age fifty (typically, they retire early). The conversation focused on the challenges of firefighters continuing to work, with respect to keeping fit and all the rest of it. This Chief Fire Officer said, "Then, of course, there's menopause." Everything went quiet. He thought to himself, "Well, that was fun. I think I'll do it again." He then repeated, "Then, of course, there's menopause."

This same man did a lot of work around gender, gender equality, and sexuality as well. He was willing to disrupt the status quo. When I went to talk to his organization, one of the first questions I was asked was, "What about transgender people and menopause?" I immediately thought, here's a forward-thinking organization because people go through gender realignment at any age. That means we're not just talking about middle-aged women. We're talking about somebody in their twenties going through gender reassignment, which triggers early menopause. In an organization where somebody can ask that as the first question, you know you're in the right place.

Tricia: Indeed. This is such a wonderful conversation. It's just amazing. Do you have thoughts that you want to share, Alexandra, or any more questions?

Alexandra: I only have gratitude. I also want to contribute something I often say in my professional context, which is that, of course, we have our prefrontal cortexes. They are wonderful for learning calculus and all kinds of other things as well. However, we are mammals, and mammals learn primarily through imitation. Especially when it comes to relationships, that is the case. Menopause is definitely one of those areas where we learn through imitation. So I'm very, very grateful that you continue to create so much around menopause that is worth imitating and that you altogether live in a way that is worthy of emulation.

Pat: I've spoken about this all around the world. I've been on stages in India, Singapore, Iceland, and more. I'm not afraid to say menstrual periods or vaginal dryness. When I name these things, it reassures women that they can talk about them too. Whether they've been through a hysterectomy or cancer treatment or they're going through menopause, it's all okay. We're women, and we can talk about all of this directly without shame. I sometimes feel my confidence and forthrightness on the subject gives others confidence too, as well as permission.

I've run a number of online courses and workshops, as well as some additional programs for an educational institution in Cambridge. I run a five-week course for them, which meets one night each week for two hours. That is ten full hours of training about menopause. Every time we run the course, I say, "I'll only take twelve people maximum." Every single time they fill up. But I only take twelve because I want to be able to see the women and talk to them intimately.

When I get to the end of the training, I ask what was the most significant thing you've learned here? So many of them say that it was so lovely to talk to other women. I used to think I might just as well open up the Zoom room and lay down for a couple of hours. But of course, it is essential that I facilitate the conversation and make the topic normal and natural, so we can talk about itchy skin and all the other symptoms with relative ease. Whether you want to take hormones, do exactly what your doctor said when you had an appointment, ignore the doctor's advice, or anything else, including how you advocated for yourself in the process, are all important considerations and worthy of conversation. The course provides women an opportunity to talk about menopause in a natural way, and that itself is highly beneficial.

Tricia: I love what you've said. So many women disparage themselves when they're going through menopause.

Pat: Absolutely. I also focus on helping them out of the mindset that menopause is somehow "the end" of the best parts of their lives. No. It's the end of a phase. But it's not "THE end." Furthermore, menopause is very much about entering into a new phase.

And guess what? It's pretty good fun in this phase! I give so many less fucks about anything. When women hear me say that, they look within and recognize that they feel similarly. I quickly hear, "Gee, you know, I don't care as much either. Wow! This is quite fantastic. You know, I'm still going to turn up looking as good as I can look. But I'm not going to spend all my time looking in the mirror wondering if I've got spots or not, or whether my eyebrows are right, or what anybody else thinks about what I've said."

Tricia: I love it.

Alexandra: It's amazing to hear this laid out so clearly, and compellingly! I have come to believe that women in our culture come to a fork in the road unconsciously. They don't necessarily recognize it's a fork in the road and a decision to make, but there is. There's the way forward that you're describing, where life gets a lot more interesting, and women become more unapologetic. Then there's the other path which many take that leads to all the disheartening statistics about being post-menopausal.

I'm so excited and inspired by how much has already been established in the UK that has normalized menopause and empowered women going through it. This is not something I've ever encountered in the US. I remember thinking, "Hmmm. Menopause in the workplace...What does that even mean?" I see now what a truly important matter it is, and it sure sounds like the UK is leading the way with your and others' influence. I'm thrilled and hopeful that there won't be too much of a lag time before people in the US begin paying attention and implementing such changes here as well.

Pat: I get more and more inquiries from all over. I did a webinar for Reuters a couple of years ago; I did one for their Pan-Pacific offices and one for their North American offices. Reuters had started publishing articles about menopause and wanted their staff to be more aware. We had about 200 people on the North American call, and they asked many questions. It was quite a lively discussion.

I met a woman, Dr. Rachel Cady, who's in Minnesota. She came to my summit yesterday to talk about hormone therapy. We really want to raise awareness and educate people. As part of this goal, Dr. Cady imparted the truth to everyone that the misinformation of women is a billion-dollar industry. There are hundreds of companies trying to get women to take things and use things that are not going to make any difference at all, or worse, they will cause harm.

Tricia: I think what you're saying is so valuable, and it has me wondering, why do we want everyone to just be fine? What about normalizing being fully inside the experience of menopause, claiming it, and using it as fuel for purpose and passion? Is it because people don't want to see someone sweating in a meeting because of a hot flash that we try to minimize that symptom? What is everyone so afraid of?

Pat: I'll respond with a story about my friend. She only lives a few doors down the street from me. We've been friends since our children were babies. She's always been very out there about whatever she's experiencing at each stage of her life. We used to go to networking meetings together, and she'd announce, "Well, hang on a minute, everybody. I'm having a hottie. I'll be alright in a minute. Just give me a second." She is an entrepreneur. She was out there doing whatever she wanted, and her attitude was, "What is the problem?"

I think she could do that partly because she's dyslexic. That might sound weird, but to this day, she makes up words. If she doesn't know a word and she needs one, she just makes up a word. If somebody challenges her, she responds by saying that the original word (the one she couldn't think of) wasn't the right word, so she provided a better one. Frequently she also points out that the person who challenged her understood what she meant, which was the point of it all. They say, "Oh, yes, I did." My friend then looks them in the eye and says, "Then what was your problem?" She's just that way and believes if someone has a problem, that's their problem, not hers. She's dealing with her stuff. She expects you to deal with yours. She's excellent that way. She just calls people out if they question her and say something is wrong. "Why? Why is it wrong?" She has brought that matter-of-factness to her menopause journey as well.

Alexandra: I love this. How you do anything is how you do everything–what a fabulous example!

Tricia: One of the things I do in the world is support people in speaking, how they use language, how they show up, and communicate effectively. What you're saying is so valuable because if your friend who says, "Hang on, I'm having a hottie," had instead framed it the way most women do, saying something like "I'm so sorry, I'm having a hot flash, excuse me," it would have been a very different communication. Right? The typical way is to camouflage the experience so no one has to witness it. But your friend's way–that's what not giving a fuck looks like! To simply say, "I am having a hot flash, which is so sexy because I'm going to have to take my shirt off right now."

Pat: Oh, yes! It makes me think of another woman I know named Susan. I met her ten or twelve years ago. She was an extremely attractive woman. I met her because she had developed a product for hot flashes. It's a kind of cold pack you can carry around with you in an insulated case.

She told me the first time she had a hot flash, she was in an office talking to a handsome younger male colleague.

She started to get a hot flash and was flicking her hair the way women sometimes do when they're having hot flashes and want to get their hair off their neck. The younger male colleague mistakenly thought she was coming on to him! Then he started flirting back. She finished her story by saying, "You know, in the end, I married him!"

Tricia: Oh, I love it. She sounds so sexy in that moment! I want more women to hear more of those stories.

Pat: A goddess, she was being a goddess in that moment. She was so funny and forthright too. I remember she was looking for an investor to finance the hot flash cooling pack she was making. She had to do research and really prepare to pitch the company. During that time, she went into a meeting with a whole bunch of financiers who were men. She explained her product and the details of its benefits. One of the men in attendance said, "I don't really get it. Why couldn't you just hold an ice cube?" She responded, "If you had erectile dysfunction, and I said to you, why don't you just use a pencil? How would you feel about it?"

Alexandra: My goodness. There's something that's so straightforward, and also quite radical, in menopause done with the authenticity of the sort you've been describing. I have found this conversation incredible. Our readers are going to love the amazing stories and be inspired by both the breadth and specificity of what you've shared.

Tricia: I feel so grateful. What you've shared is just so important. I have never worked in a company, and I know

Alexandra hasn't for a long time either. This makes us especially appreciative to hear your point of view and include it in this conversation. Thank you for sharing what you're doing for the workplace–learning about your projects has been fascinating.

chapter 6
REDEFINING MENOPAUSE

Tricia: So much to digest with Pat, right?

Alexandra: So much. It's shifted my thinking about possible titles for our book. Now I'm considering *Evolution and Identity: Welcome To Menopause* or *Evolution and Identity: Your Invitation to Menopause.*

Tricia: I like that: A welcome or an invitation. It also reflects my invitation to you to co-author this book. When we invite one another to talk about menopause, to share in this diverse experience together, we de-stigmatize it. It's taking away the idea that menopause is something scary. Instead, it's something to go to, to show up for, like a gala.

Alexandra: Ha, yes. Exactly. Welcome to the party.

Tricia: So, in terms of the conversation with Pat...is there anything you want to discuss?

Alexandra: Well, I'm still pondering the tendency to pathologize menopause. Her response to my question about that was to compare it to adolescence. But when it comes to adolescence, there isn't a big gender distinction. Boys' voices drop, and they develop muscles. Girls develop breasts and start menstruating. To be more precise, there's a big gender distinction, but adolescence impacts everybody in one way or another. Even so, there is no denying that the meaningful, empowering opportunities inherent in both puberty and menopause are often dismissed. "Oh, it's just puberty. You'll get through it."

Tricia: I think you are right about things being more gender equal in puberty than they are in menopause, probably because males go through puberty too.

Do you think men go through a kind of menopause—their own, albeit subtler version of it?

Alexandra: Well, men certainly go through midlife crises, which can be both subtle or rather overt. I am not sure if that is similar to what we are talking about or not—at first glance, it doesn't appear so.

Tricia: I really want to look up the origin of the word "menopause" to see what it reveals.

Alexandra: Oh, yes!

Tricia: Okay, wow, so menopause literally means the end of monthly cycles. It comes from the Greek word "men," meaning month, and "pause," meaning end. So literally, the simplest and most appropriate definition of menopause is the end of monthly cycles. That's all. No more periods, period.

Alexandra: That reflects exactly what Pat was talking about when it comes to treating menopause as a biological phenomenon rather than an opportunity to shed former identities and step into a new glorious one.

Tricia: Yes. It also says the word is derived from the French, a word meaning the final cessation of monthly courses of women. Wow. So it's basically the end of you, right? You have ceased.

Alexandra: It's as if, once your fertility is over, your function as a person has been served. Everything afterward is just dead weight.

Tricia: Exactly.

Alexandra: Now I'm wondering what the etymology of the word "puberty" is!

Tricia: I'll find it. It says "puberty" is from the Latin word meaning adult. So the word "puberty" seems to be about where you are heading.

That is a big difference! Menopause reflects the ending, and puberty points to the new beginning.

Alexandra: Okay, well, at this point, that feels more like a confirmation than a surprise, meaning that distinction reflects the dominant attitude in society. If I take it to an extreme, it practically implies viewing menopause treatment as if it's palliative care. It's whacko because it's clear there is so much potential for what is possible on the other side of menopause—it really doesn't feel accurate to characterize menopause by endings alone. Plus, these days, more and more people live longer than they ever have before.

Tricia: It's true.

Alexandra: I want the experiences we talk about here, along with the experiences of other women, to create a sense of belonging so that no one feels like an outlier. I want everyone to know that when it comes to menopause, the experience is part of what it means to be human, for women anyway. This is not a kind of termination diagnosis but rather an invitation to whatever is next.

Tricia: Wouldn't it be cool if people even looked forward to menopause? I find myself wondering if the absence of anticipatory worry would have expedited my evolution; if a book like the one we're working on had existed when I went off the pill at fifty-one, I may not have been so concerned about what was coming.

Alexandra: That's wonderful to consider, and there is something important about charting your own path that specifically enhances it. There are many anecdotal reports of various medical miracles where people go into remission or are able to cure themselves in ways that fly in the face of accepted scientific practice. Norman Cousins is a great example of this. He locked himself in a hotel room with many comedies and basically laughed away his terminal illness. When other people subsequently watched a lot of comedies and laughed extensively, they didn't necessarily have extraordinary healing. Or similarly, someone does a green juice fast for cancer, goes into remission, tells other people about it, and then they do green juice fasts too. But those people do not reliably go into remission. No treatment or modality or outcome is a one size fits all solution, but it seems that trusting oneself and writing one's own script is important when going off the beaten path.

I'm wanting to point out, when it comes to health and healing, that there's something important about being internally free enough to do something your own way. When someone has conviction and goes fully and courageously into an experience, being willing to follow their own instincts and trust the process is as important as the particular treatments or activities carried out. So maybe it would have been easier for you if you had read our book before getting to menopause, but I also think it's significant that you forged your own path with such clarity and boldness.

In this context, I'll state my desire for this book to be an inspiration and to serve to open people's minds to what is possible. But also, I do not want to encourage anyone to do as I have done or as you have done. Just because it worked for each of us doesn't mean anything about how it will work for someone else. When it comes to shedding old identities and stepping into new ones or managing physical symptoms, it's quite clear that there isn't a universal recipe. I imagine you would wholeheartedly agree with me.

Tricia: Exactly, I do. I also want to emphasize this point because the very nature of menopause has so much to do with finding your own unique voice or experience. I hope this book serves to inspire and give permission to other women to also share their experiences, whatever they are.

We want to articulate the potential transformation, purpose, and alignment newly available in menopause. That's the transmission. But this is not a roadmap instructing people what to do. Ultimately people have to choose for themselves whether or not to befriend the changes that are happening, or not, and see where it goes.

Alexandra: I love that distinction so much. I would underline it, highlight it, and put it in bold. You're right; it's not a roadmap. A roadmap feels too masculine and too linear for what we're talking about anyway. That has its place, but there is no defined destination here. Women can craft their own. It's not just Grandma Moses whose career started at seventy-eight! Many other women have made incredible contributions, both personally and professionally, after menopause. I don't know when the cultural narrative around menopause began to equate menopause with the beginning of the end, but it's done us all a major disservice.

I am menopausal and feel incredibly far from over the hill! I have not peaked. Okay, well, I've peaked with respect to childbearing. I haven't peaked in motherhood. I haven't peaked at learning new things or serving others in meaningful ways. I haven't peaked when it comes to having fun or pleasure either. There is so much more fantastic life that awaits me. The idea that after thirty-five, it's all downhill is so far from my actual experience.

Saying I'm menopausal, which I've never said before today, needs to feel authentic. I'm finding there's a toxic residue on the phrase that I want to remove. The implied dehydration the word "menopause" carries for me is rather unappealing. I didn't realize I felt this strongly about it until having this conversation, but now I'm not surprised that I didn't identify as menopausal.

Tricia: What you're talking about is so big. There are huge implications associated with menopause that are present in our society. This attitude is passed down to us even before we begin to experience physiological changes. Having the opportunity to talk as we are, making use of our voices, platforms, and our very essence, is intended to redefine menopause and contribute more positive associations. I hope we update the dialogue.

We are living our menopause experiences, sharing them honestly. Doing so may contribute to preventing menopause from being largely associated with dehydration and assorted limitations.

Alexandra: Yes, what is commonly believed is often confused with what is true. This is a situation where they definitely are not the same.

I am imagining a future in which someone creates something akin to "The Vagina Monologues" focused on menopause.

The monologues resulted in the word "vagina" becoming far more commonplace in US households, and I can imagine something similar when it comes to menopause.

Tricia: Right. Culturally imposed ideas about menopause tell us once it comes, we're over. That has nothing to do with biological phenomena.

Alexandra: It is definitely not related to biological phenomena; well, I suppose it is in terms of the word menopause describing the cessation of menses. But after menopause comes so much else that isn't conveyed in the word "menopause."

Tricia: Yes. Maybe we don't need to redefine or rename it. But we do need to show up in a different way when it comes to menopause. I think what you're saying is very true. I mean, if I get up in the morning, look at myself in the mirror, and say, "Good Morning, I'm in menopause," it feels weird. However, the reality is that I am in menopause, and physiologically, I am no longer able to have children. But none of that means I'm "less than" or stopping anything. The fact that I'm in menopause also does not mean that I'm invisible, dead, or ending as a person, as the word seems to imply.

Alexandra: When I was forty-two and living in southwest rural Kansas, I was at a meeting with other women, where each of us introduced ourselves. We went around the room with each person saying what they do. There was one woman who said, "I'm a mother," with conviction, clarity, pride, and a sense of completeness. It made a huge impression on me because I realized I'd never experienced that before. For me, being a mother has always been quite wonderful, while also totally inadequate and incomplete as a description of who I am.

Throughout my adulthood, I've had many identities reflecting my accomplishments, such as student, doctor, homeowner, teacher, etc. I discovered an unconscious belief in me that said if I didn't include any accomplishments beyond motherhood in my introduction, no one would pay attention to what I had to say. In other words, being a mother was not enough to command the room. When I heard this woman say she was a mother (as a complete identity), it impacted me. It showed me I could relate to my identity as a mother far more fully because, in that moment, I understood that being a mother didn't need accessorizing.

Similarly, through the conversations encapsulated in this book, I want to embody a different relationship to menopause so that when I say, "I am menopausal," it feels both accurate and exciting.

Tricia: This is good. I think the reason so many women are afraid to talk about menopause is because they are afraid that their entire identities will be reduced to this one thing.

Alexandra: Yes, and yet, there is scientific research showing that cultures where postmenopausal women are revered as important elders tend to function successfully and enjoy longevity. Unsurprisingly, women in these cultures fare a great deal better than women in cultures where postmenopausal women are not revered and are essentially overlooked.

When considering how many older women in our culture feel invisible and, by inference, irrelevant, let's keep in mind that the expected lifespan of humans has almost doubled. This means the experience of being postmenopausal and being postmenopausal for decades is a fairly new phenomenon in human history.

Tricia: Yes, so why would we let it be defined for us at all?

Alexandra: Right?

Doctors define menopause as the time when a woman has not had a period for 12 consecutive months. Then a woman is postmenopausal. "Postmenopausal," as I understand it, refers to the time after menopause has been completed. Technically, a woman is postmenopausal from the day menopause occurs until the end of her life.

In casual language, it sounds as if menopause is just like menarche, the name for a girl's first period. But in reality, menopause is nothing like menarche. Menarche is a one-time event. You know when it is happening. You know when it's completed. In contrast, menopause is a process that feels like it lasts several years; it's certainly hard to know precisely when it starts or when it will end.

Tricia: So, the word "postmenopausal" doesn't really make sense because what we're actually doing is experiencing sustained menopause.

Alexandra: Yes, there is no "beyond menopause" unless you are no longer alive. Probably, medically speaking, the phrase is used because the transition has been completed. Even so, in terms of a literal definition, it makes no sense.

Tricia: What's interesting to me is how menopause is talked about as something to be endured. Even Pat Duckworth said, "You'll get to the other side." So is the other side being postmenopausal? I guess so. Your brain fog goes away, your clarity comes back, the hot flashes stop, and then there you are…you're postmenopausal.

Alexandra: That sounds so apocalyptic.

Tricia: It does.

Again, part of what we're doing here is trying to get people to talk about things openly and authentically, differently than before, so we can see menopause isn't a sort of punishment or sentence. Right?

Alexandra: Absolutely. The conversation can be awkward and confusing, too personal, or amazing and empowered, and we are here for all of it. Because it's all true.

Is there anything else that came up for you during our talk with Pat?

Tricia: Well, one thing is that I was just so moved by her generosity. She's a stranger to us. She's written five books, she's an expert, and she's willing to share so much. I find that she's mirroring our own conversations and affirming this is really how the sisterhood of menopause operates.

Alexandra: Yes, the sisterhood of menopause. The sisterhood of women who are real with themselves and see much more is possible, both individually and in each area of our life, including business.

I really loved her mastery. You're used to having mastery and witnessing it with your clients. I'm used to having it and witnessing it with my clients and various other aspects of my life, but it was new and so wonderfully rich to experience mastery in the context of menopause and the related issues, including identity.

Tricia: Yes. I want to name that I feel really full, not so full that there isn't room for more, but I feel so nourished. The whole conversation really sparked my imagination.

Alexandra: I understand. As we've been speaking, both with Pat and just the two of us, I was thinking I'd like to have a conversation like this with you every few years. It doesn't need to lead to a book being published. It could, but that's not required! The fact that we're speaking now in order to create a book definitely enhances this conversation deeply. But the whole weekend of focused discussions is transformative in its own right. It's created an intentional sisterhood between us. This flavor of sisterhood is something I want more of in my life because it's an attitude. It's a way of being. It's an invitation to both go within and come out for connection.

Another way to put it is that I feel initiated now.

Tricia: Alexandra, I'm so glad that we are doing this together and that we trust each other deeply enough to be open to what transpires. As I said earlier, I never would have wanted to do a book project with anyone else. I've never done something like this before, and I find it's really, really, special work. I'm just so grateful. I'm so grateful for Pat, but also so grateful for you.

Alexandra: I feel the same way. Something has really opened up through the deliciousness of extended conversation and the ways we set it up from the outset.

But what is it that you feel you've never done before?

Tricia: That's such a great question. I've never intentionally created a womb like this in my home for creative activity with someone else. I've always been alone. Doing it together feels expansive and powerful. The intentionality that I have brought to every detail has been part of this creative process for me, and it's been full of joy.

The other part is our being so honest and vulnerable about something nobody else talks about. That is definitely something I've never done before. I've spoken to Joe about menopause and a couple of friends. But knowing that I am doing it with you feels safe. It also feels risky, which is a good thing. Even just with you, never having been to my home before and not likely to have if we weren't choosing to engage in this way. Now, through this process, we've both said yes to and co-created we have a relationship that's extremely intimate without knowing a whole lot about each other beyond what we know professionally.

Alexandra: Well, yes, that's a good point. It's making me realize that I have a belief I wasn't aware of until this moment. I've become aware that I previously thought this kind of collaboration is more likely to occur when there's already a deep personal connection, which is then transferred or extended into the professional realm. But we are an example of taking a professional connection and intentionally transitioning it into such a personal collaboration. The result has incredible potency and depth.

Add to this that, in the past, I always thought of myself as someone who doesn't collaborate well. I have had good collaborations before, but I definitely don't seek them out, and the times I've enjoyed most are when each person's role is very well defined. That allows me to attend to my roles and responsibilities in my own way, without the complications associated with having someone involved who is not aligned with my vision or not showing up the way I would like.

That's how it was when I hosted you for the Speakers Salon in San Francisco. I did things my way, and you did things your way. I took care of finding a venue, enrolling students, and handling logistics, and had nothing whatsoever to do with the content which was entirely provided by you. My contribution provided the support for you to present brilliantly, and I was thrilled to be your student during the event. That's a totally different dynamic than this one, where we are both discovering what's next and communicating accordingly.

I believe the personal growth we've each done in our lives is what allows for this level of honesty because you would never want to participate without honesty, and I wouldn't either. We need this level of honesty and trust for what we're creating.

Tricia: Yes, and one more thing I want to highlight is that you are exactly who you are. I don't ever have to worry you're going to become someone else. I hope you understand what that means, or I can try to explain it if you'd like me to.

Alexandra: Please explain it as it may be a place that I naturally have a blind spot because, well, I only know myself as myself, and it feels like a very important point.

Tricia: To put it plainly, I have a deep trust in you because you show up consistently. You are clear about who you are. You're clear about what your point of view is, and I trust you're not going to all of a sudden become someone else, which would end up shifting the foundation we've established. I have a lot of trust in my relationships; however, I find that sometimes people aren't always consistent, and not everyone has the same level of integrity, not of the quality I see in you.

Alexandra: Thank you for that reflection.

Tricia: We began this co-creation after you said, "Yes, and let me think about it." Then each of us went off on our own to think about it. We considered it. "Okay, this is a great idea." "We want to collaborate, but what does that look like?" "What does that feel like?" Only then did we come back to the next call with "This is what I would like," "That is what I would like." We didn't even discuss if it was going to be in

New York. You just said, "I'll come to New York." And that felt wonderful. It wasn't something I had expected.

I want to acknowledge this kind of synergy isn't always going to be present, and it's not required. I'm hoping our book will inspire readers to think about what it might mean for them to co-create in any aspect of their lives.

Alexandra: I like that. It can be a transmission of what's possible, a transmission of multi-layered truths. We're not trying to sell menopause as this amazing fabulous thing. We're just telling the truth about what it can be and what it has been for us as we redefine it and locate it in our lives right now.

Tricia: Oh, another title idea just came to me: *Menopause: A Reclamation*

Alexandra: Oh yes, that is good, a definite contender.

chapter 7

IMPORTANT SHIFTS

Tricia: I don't know if this has to do with menopause specifically, but I notice my husband has been even more of a participant in our family–the family that includes him and I, our cats, and what is important to us. Our marriage is so much deeper and richer now. He is so different from how he was ten years ago. I think this is so interesting because even though a woman's eggs are no longer viable in menopause, and she is no longer fertile when it comes to the possibility of biological children, women are still vessels of creation and transformation. Maybe that's part of menopause–a turning away from one type of creation towards another.

Alexandra: I have that experience with my husband, Rodd, too.

I see a relationship between menopause and the notion of a midlife crisis. But "midlife crisis" often evokes impulsive actions like buying a new red sports car or having an affair.

What if this same crisis energy, instead of splitting up marriages or emptying bank accounts, could instead be directed or redirected with incredibly positive results, bringing in more aliveness and passion and deepening a man's sense of purpose.

In Rodd's case, he began talking about wanting to switch from very full-time doctor hours to working part-time. He's the Chief of his department and had the option to continue in that role while working fewer hours and for less pay. When he'd bring up this possibility, I would feel anxious. There's very little I get anxious about when it comes to discussing future plans and possibilities; however, it happened every time he brought up this topic. On the other hand, this was what he wanted. Still, it was very triggering for me every time he would speak about it. I had financial concerns because working fewer hours would mean he would be making less money. I also worried that dialing down his hours would be a way he would withdraw from life. I thought working less might turn him into an old man or that he would be dialing down his sense of contribution to our lives. Something about this felt emotionally unsafe for me. It wasn't logical; however, it was real.

Nevertheless, in 2019 he decided to move forward with his plans and only told me after he had arranged the transition. I was supportive and quite upset, although I tried to hide it. At one point, my resentment came flying out, and I said, "You know, it's not about the decision, but that you made it yourself. We didn't decide together. That's not how we navigate important choices. I really don't like that you didn't include me." He responded carefully, saying, "I wanted to talk with you, but I couldn't. You refused to have that conversation with me." I immediately saw he was right; I wouldn't have that conversation. In my refusal to discuss it, I left him no choice but to suffer or make a decision without me. Once I comprehended that, I wasn't upset anymore. I understood that he really had tried to connect about it, and I was completely unavailable for a discussion. Anyway, the plan was in place, and he transitioned to working three days a week.

Tricia: Three days a week! Did that schedule end up being amazing for your relationship?

Alexandra: Well, eventually, but I want to emphasize two things. One is that this whole thing was very complicated for him to navigate in the context of our marriage. It wasn't easy for him to honor what he wanted to do on his own, but I wasn't available to participate in what would have otherwise been a collaborative decision for us. I think that felt lonely for him.

Furthermore, something about such a big change, even if I wasn't the one making it, was unnerving for me. I'm trying to convey that I resisted his evolving identity. I'm not proud of that, although the point here is that men also can evolve in beautiful ways in this phase of life, and the people who love them may not support them (which, in this case, was me).

In terms of your question about whether it was amazing for our relationship, I would say yes, but it took some time to get there.

Tricia: How so?

Alexandra: Well, at first, we navigated some new power dynamics. You see, I'd been making meals, homeschooling, figuring out the driving, the shopping, and all the household things for our family for twenty-one years. I had been working, but I always ran our household and oversaw our children's schooling and other needs. Rodd was a loving father for sure, very supportive and hands-on when available, but he used to work so many hours. This meant that I carried a tremendous amount of our family and household responsibilities, and relatively speaking, he was uninvolved. Once he was home four days a week, and I worked three of them, there were a lot of new experiences and new discoveries for both of us.

For example, for a good year, Rodd was unable to wash the dishes at the same time he was attending to our children. He just couldn't do both. It was too overwhelming for him. So our house was a mess. In addition, on the days he had committed to caring for our children while I worked more, I would emerge from my home office and find that dinner wasn't ready and he hadn't even thought about it.

I had a lot of judgment about him being unreliable and unsupportive. I had been handling all these things for years, and it wasn't challenging for me to make it all happen. It had been challenging initially, but that was so long ago when we had babies in diapers, and I was nursing, along with attending to all the tasks and responsibilities. Anyway, so many years later, I took it for granted that I could engage with our elementary and high school-aged children, cook dinner, and schedule a dentist appointment during the course of two hours without it being a big deal. But he was unable to.

At first, I considered it kind of pathetic until I understood that actually, being with children in such a hands-on way is a skill that grows with practice. Then, rather than looking down at him, I began to value what I had done. I had done it without a second thought for many years, and for the first time, I began to appreciate my contribution to our family more thoroughly. Seeing how challenging this transition was for him gave me a window into my own power, my own capabilities, and also my ability to love.

Another important part of this transition was not just Rodd's growth; it also included the monumental challenge for me to learn how to let go of control. He needed the space to do things his own way, without me micromanaging or expecting he would do things the same way I did in every aspect of parenting and tending our household. Honestly, I now see that he does many things better than I did. I wouldn't have discovered that without making room within me to be relaxed while he went through trial and error and a sustained level of chaos we hadn't had to deal with in years. Learning to let go and also trust him with our family matters has expanded me in wonderful ways and been absolutely amazing for our relationship. This, even more than having more time together, has wonderfully evolved the culture of our marriage.

At the same time, this created space for me to dive into my own work with a robustness and devotion that has been thrilling for me. In terms of it being amazing for our relationship, the thing I would say is that I now feel profoundly supported in a way I had never known. I never knew I could truly let go of family and household matters and be fully present in pursuing my own purpose. It's hard to describe but suffice it to say, I never knew this level of support was available until I began to experience it. These days he does all the interactions with the other moms for our son's baseball team. He makes sure the kids have new sneakers when they need them and another tube of toothpaste when the old one runs out. These sound like minor things, but emotional labor piles up.

Nowadays, if I feel like cooking dinner when he's with the children, then I do. But if I don't feel like it, then I don't need to think about it because he will. Plus, my ability to immerse myself in my own work is so much deeper than it ever was before because I don't need to have so much ambient attention on my children. I've tapped into a reservoir of creativity, conviction, and clarity in how I serve couples that I just couldn't have accessed before because I had to keep some attention on my kids or be available if one of them needed something. So, on the one hand, I have passion and purpose that I associate with the new energy available in menopause, and on the other, my ability to act on it and go deep is very much contextualized by Rodd's choice. We've both benefited immensely from his shifting from having a strong career identity to one of a devoted hands-on father and outstanding partner.

Tricia: Wow, I can only imagine.

Alexandra: The way things are now has always been my vision for how we would be as our children leave home, but I really didn't know how the heck we would get here. I'm curious if you have a way that you've oriented to or anticipated this phase beyond what we've already covered.

Tricia: I think it has to do with maturity. It feels like there is a strong correlation between maturity and menopause. You and I happen to be in very, very solid, loving marriages, so that's the point of view we're speaking from. If I were dating at this time of my life, I think I would feel a freedom that I did not experience prior to being married when I was dating.

Alexandra: That is definitely true for me as well.

Currently, the highest percentage of divorce is among couples who've been married for thirty years or longer, meaning people who are in their fifties, sixties, and seventies want something different. Perhaps the idea that it's mostly women who have to cope with the challenges of menopause on their own isn't as true as it used to be because their men are quite affected too. I'll add that, in my opinion, for most men, it's definitely not too late, at fifty or sixty, to learn to be genuinely connected with their partner. And when your partner is in menopause, it's a great time to cultivate that skill!

Tricia: Yes, I would agree. Even men who are very evolved and self-aware have much to learn about this phase of life.

chapter 8
MENOPAUSE AND PARTNERSHIP

Tricia: I'm curious if you've had a conversation with Rodd about this project or about menopause in general? I know Rodd knows you're here with me in New York City in order to write this book, but what else?

Joe is so excited! He has been supportive and involved with the idea from the beginning. When I shared my hot flashes in real time with Joe and how I felt about taking my health into my own hands, in his charming comedic way, he threw out, "You should write a book about what to expect when you're sweating." That was a whole year before I reached out to you. I had to sit with it.

Alexandra: I love that title. I laughed so hard when you shared that with me.

And no, I haven't had an explicit conversation with Rodd about menopause. I realized that when we were speaking earlier. It just hasn't seemed relevant, and it never occurred to me. I mean, right now, in this conversation with you, I'm seeing how relevant it actually is. Probably it's been relevant before, but I hadn't been seeing my life, my marriage, or really anything at all through the lens of menopause, so I didn't bring it up. He didn't either.

Tricia: How does it feel to have menopause become relevant as a lens, specifically in your marriage?

Alexandra: Well, let's see, there's a lot of context to share before I answer because the scene was set long ago.

I grew up in a family that never used anatomical, cutesy, or even euphemistic language for female genitalia. I have no memory of when I learned anatomical terms, but I was definitely in my teens. This sounds like something from another century, but I was born in 1968. My mother was a very educated woman (while also being a hippie from the 1960s). She certainly knew her anatomy and knew how to use all parts of it, but she didn't transmit this knowledge to me. I didn't know the word vagina. I didn't know the words pussy, yoni, or coochie, either. I didn't actually discuss sex with my mother until I'd already had two children. I used to be really angry about that, but I've come to perceive the love in my mother's choices. My grandmother was very expressive and said all kinds of things about her body and her feelings, etc. As a child, my mother found that overwhelming to take in. She didn't want me to have to navigate that. She wanted to give me space to develop naturally, so to speak, so she chose to say nothing about a lot of things.

In high school, I had very bad menstrual cramps. I missed days of school because I was experiencing heavy bleeding, intense cramps, and sometimes needed to vomit. It wasn't every month, but it was often enough. Only after this had been going on for years did my mother share with me that she had experienced the same kind of periods in high school as had her mother, my grandmother. She told me that my grandmother talked about her periods in such dramatic terms, and my mother had wondered if her own physical symptoms were the result of her mother's projections and her own suggestibility. She hoped that if she never spoke about how intense menstruation had been for her, I would be spared the experience of comparable physical symptoms. Never speaking about it was intended to spare me suffering, though it turned out not to matter whether she had told me or not.

Tricia: This is so interesting.

Alexandra: Jumping ahead, I met Rodd in the first week of medical school. In the first ten years of our relationship, while dating and then marriage, we were both working super long hours. We often worked sixty or up to one hundred hours per week. During this time, I had one child while in medical school and one just before my internship began. Our early years were defined by babies in diapers and lots and lots of work. During this time, our love grew, and our communication skills blossomed, but our sex wasn't anything like what the poets write about. I definitely did not feel a sense of communion, of the merging of our souls, of tapping into a wellspring of pleasure. We both assumed that once we had more time with one another, then our intimate life would organically evolve and become more enlivened and gratifying.

Ten years down the road, we had our weekends off, we had our evenings together, and we didn't have any little children. But once we had time together, the flavors of our intimacy never really changed that much. That's when we learned it wasn't just time that we had lacked. We needed education, connection, and so much more. We needed reinvention.

Learning how to ignite the passion in our marriage was part of what inspired me to become a Relationship and Intimacy Coach, so I can teach others how to turn on their relationships, sex lives, and life!

All of that is context for me to say that I now see having a conversation about menopause—both the physical symptoms and the existential invitation—to be an essential part of reclamation, embodiment, and vulnerable, honest, passion-fueling intimacy in midlife and beyond.

Tricia: When Joe and I decided to get married, we opted to be married by a Zen Buddhist priestess. She was amazing. She was in San Francisco at the Zen Center. When we talked with her about it, she said, "Okay, and I want to support you by coaching you for a year before you get married so that you can both be on the same page when you get married." We did a year of coaching with her. In addition, we went to couples counseling. We loved our therapist, and I would highly recommend them. However, in every session with our therapist, Joe and I talked about all that was wrong with the week, the relationship, or both. Keep in mind this was before we were even married. We continued therapy for a long time after being married as well. We looked at it as a kind of maintenance for us.

Then my dad died. He had Parkinson's and, in the end, was in hospice. It was the first time either one of us had lost a parent. I didn't know I was going to respond the way I did because I had never lost a parent. But it was a big, big identity shift for me. I found myself asking, "Who am I now?" "Who do I need to be now?" "Who do I want to be now?" "How am I going to relate to my mother now?" "How will everything be?"

During this time, I kept finding Joe wrong. He was not who I wanted him to be. It just…something felt impossible, and I was frustrated. I remember waking up one morning, the day after we'd gone to therapy, saying to myself, "Fuck this. This is not working." I knew it wasn't on him; it was on me. I was changing. I had to change. I knew I couldn't ask him to be different, to change who he was. That's not my role. Instead, I have to focus on myself; I'm the one who needs to change.

I eventually realized I didn't need him to be anything or anyone other than exactly who he is. Whatever I needed, I needed to be that for myself. I loosened my grip and let go. I shifted the energy. I said, "Honey, therapy isn't working for me anymore. I would like to do a family meeting instead." He just turned to me and asked, "What does that mean? What's a family meeting?" We sat down at the kitchen table, and I told him everything that I loved about him and all the wonderful things that had taken place during the week prior. He was so surprised because he was waiting for the bad stuff.

Alexandra: Did he think he might be in trouble?

Tricia: Yes. But I wasn't upset. What I wanted was to have a positive, affirming time together.

I said to him, "My only request from you is that we have a family meeting every Saturday at four o'clock, every single Saturday." He promptly agreed. I then said, "Honey, I love you. Here's what is amazing about you, and here's what's amazing about us." Afterward, he shared too. He started sharing in a way that was so different from what was happening in therapy, and I loved it. We started to actually communicate. No more rehashing of all the crap we didn't do well.

It was a complete shift in energy. To this day, if it's 3:59 PM on a Saturday, and I'm in the other room, he will come in and say, "It's time for the family meeting." We then sit down and share with one another in these ways. He sits in that chair you're in right now, and I sit in my chair here. Afterward, we get up. We stand right here and hug and kiss. We started about seven years into our marriage, and it has created this consistent, beautiful thing that's been going on for years now. It happens every Saturday. The family meeting has created a complete energetic shift for us. It required me to change my own energy, which involved shedding the belief that I am a victim of his shortcomings.

Alexandra: I totally get it. It's really amazing.

When I start coaching couples, in the first session, I almost always ask, "How did you fall in love with one another? What was it?" Or "What do you love about one another?" Almost 100 percent of the time, people say things that their spouse didn't know previously–it's just never come up in conversation before. Interestingly, it's often related to whatever is challenging in the relationship.

I have been coaching a couple, where he feels frustrated because she is constantly asking more of him. He feels pressure to keep growing and evolving. He also felt she would never be satisfied, no matter what he did, no matter how far he came. In another context, it came out that one of the things he found most attractive about her is the way she's always bringing new things to the table. She innovates and explores. She's a curious and enthusiastic person, and he loves how it enriches life for both of them.

When he focused on what attracted him to her, their dynamic shifted. It was true that she would never be satisfied, but that was just who she was. He didn't need to take it personally when she had her eyes on their next form of advancement. Instead of seeing her drive to grow and improve as being a drawback, he came to see that being with her makes for a richer, more adventurous life. He stopped resisting, they stopped arguing, and they also started doing yoga together, taking trips, and trying different cuisines. He loves that she makes life so much more interesting for both of them.

If I hadn't asked them what had them fall in love with one another, she never would have known how he felt. She knew he was challenged by her, but not how much he cherished those same qualities. Starting with what's working is a very simple pivot, and most couples focus on what's not working without coming to that on their own.

Tricia, what you shared is brilliant. It reminds me of so many couples I have coached and how they felt about therapy. Your family meeting format is really quite special. Do you do it literally every single Saturday?

Tricia: We're very consistent. We also made a decision that we never have a family meeting if either of us has had a glass of wine. There is something else we do that we call "Threes." We ask each other, "What are three things you appreciate about yourself? What are three things you're grateful for? And what are three things you love about me?" Hearing him tell me what he appreciates about himself is very tender. Hearing how much of a good brother he is or that he appreciates how well he takes care of our girls, Lola and Bella, is so beautiful and heartwarming. I learn something new about him every single time.

He always makes me laugh because he says, "When you tell me three things you love about me, they're usually about you." I laugh and say, "What do you mean?" in a flirtatious tone.

Alexandra: Tricia, I love knowing these things. I really do.

I am continually inspired by how much is possible in our lives and in our relationships just by using the ingredients each of us already has!

Tricia: Oh, my goodness, this was the perfect day, and this is a perfect time to pause until tomorrow.

chapter 9
WALKING SCRAPBOOKS

Alexandra: Good Morning Tricia! Guess what?

Tricia: What?

Alexandra: I brought some statistics for us to consider.

Tricia: Cool!

Alexandra: Okay, here goes. Contrary to popular belief, research shows that women do not peak sexually at the age of thirty-five. Instead, for women who are sexually active, the peak occurs decades later, in their sixties and seventies. Only twelve percent of women over fifty years of age feel satisfied with their bodies, and (here's a big one) approximately fifty percent of women over age fifty are not having sex. So while it is true that many women stop having sex, paradoxically, it is also true that sexual satisfaction increases with age.

Tricia: That's incredible.

Alexandra: It is!

Tricia: So if you are a woman who is satisfied with your body, and also sexually active, and also, say, sixty-five years old, you could potentially, even scientifically, be having a really good time?

Alexandra: Yes, that is correct.

Once again, I am orienting to the phenomenon of women coming to a mostly unconscious fork in the road. People who feel badly about their bodies take one path. They stop having sex, resigned to sacrificing that part of their life. When women enjoy their bodies, it leads them in another direction, with more passion and pleasure. Of course, feeling satisfied with your body is not the only factor contributing to whether or not you're having sex. Pain, low libido, shame, lack of connection, menopausal symptoms, illness, and other contributing factors are relevant. But putting aside the cause, the data shows that approximately fifty percent of women over age fifty are no longer having sex. But for those who are, it gets better and better and better.

Tricia: Wow.

Alexandra: Relationships are such a profound arena for personal growth because the quality of our primary relationship is influenced by the quality of our communication, presence, sex (whether it's happening or not), body image, and bodily function.

I find women typically hold two beliefs about their sexuality–sometimes, the beliefs are explicit and sometimes unconscious. The first is that a woman who is menstruating should be having great sex–not necessarily while she is actively menstruating but during that time in her life. Her partner should know how to give her a great sexual experience. And secondly, a woman who is menopausal expects not to have great sex. She believes that because she is older, the sex just automatically becomes less appealing and potentially painful, and everything becomes constricted. She closes down and doesn't expect her lover to level up to make things better. She attributes challenges in the bedroom to herself, her inability to access what she used to sexually. Whereas very often, the menstruating woman might think there's something wrong with her, she also tends to think there's something wrong with her lover's technique. The menopausal/postmenopausal woman more typically thinks the challenges with sex are her "fault." I often encounter those attitudes in my work, though I consider both of them to be false narratives.

Tricia: Do you specifically address menopause with your clients?

Alexandra: Thus far, it hasn't come up that much with my clients. Couples seek me out to improve communication and/or expand their erotic experiences. I haven't found menopause to be a phase of life when couples seek me out, though it clearly could be.

For the most part, in my professional life (apart from coaching clients), I encounter menopause in one of two unappealing ways. Either it's a clinical topic that's very dry and scientific, or menopause is energetically synonymous with whining, complaining, and suffering. The meme is that menopause functions like a dictator making life miserable for the women who are affected by it.

Tricia: Given these statistics, I wonder who a sixty-five-year-old woman would be dating? I've heard about women in menopause dating men in their twenties who may not be interested in having children yet. This makes sense to me because women in menopause are no longer fertile, and it's also possible that some women in menopause are not interested in having serious relationships, so it's a perfect mix.

Alexandra: This reminds me of Pat's story about the woman having the hot flash and the young man responding to it such that they ended up marrying.

Tricia: I take my health extremely seriously. Another thing I decided when I turned fifty-one was to become younger. I decided I would not age in the traditional way. When it came to my personal mindset around aging, youth, and vitality, I would reverse time. I have a lot left to accomplish in my life. I want to write more books. Through my work, I want to help amplify and elevate as many voices as possible across the globe. I don't want to experience fatigue. I take supplements. I don't take any medications. I get a physical every year. I get regular mammograms. I am all about preventative medicine. I have extensive blood work, so I know exactly what's going on in my body, not just hormonally, as we already discussed, but for my overall health.

I'm obsessed with optimization. I have started doing cryotherapy, where I stand in a box (well, it's basically like a meat locker without meat) that's 165 degrees below zero for three minutes. I do this every week. I also stand on a bed of nails every day. Optimizing my health is very important to me. I think having this health mindset has contributed to how well I'm doing at this time in my life.

Do you want to speak to that as well?

Alexandra: Sure.

First of all, most of the sentences you just said are not true for me. I know for sure that I am not doing cryotherapy or standing on a bed of nails, but also, I haven't committed to my health the way you have. I don't have many unhealthy habits, but I haven't explicitly prioritized my health either. For me, the journey has been much more about learning to honor myself. Until fairly recently, my main functions were as a nurturer and a caretaker–along with the satisfaction and good in that, there have been challenges.

With each of my pregnancies, I gained weight after giving birth. The expectation is that after birth, one loses weight, but that's not how it was for me. There are hormonal considerations, of course, but I also attribute it to having my focus on my family's well-being and not on my own. That impacted what I ate, how I slept, whether I had time to work out and many other variables. My point is that prioritizing myself has been something I've needed to learn more recently.

Actually, during the pandemic, I lost 40 pounds, and it created an interesting shift in my identity. Surprisingly, the weight was easy to lose. We know that it's often much harder for women to lose weight around menopause, but it's been easier for me in the context of having more time, more energy, and more attention on my own well-being.

Tricia: What do you think your identity shift is about?

Alexandra: I'm not sure yet. I do know that in the past when I would go below a certain number on the scale, two days later, I would gain it back. I couldn't get below some invisible barrier. The way I think about it is that I'm essentially a walking scrapbook. There are emotions and unresolved experiences I'm holding on to from the past, and while I have largely put those things out of my mind, they have still been with me in my flesh–literally. Recently I have been journaling and paying more attention to some inner voices I've previously overridden. Doing so, coupled with some nutritional improvements, is really working for me.

I'll add that I don't have any diagnoses other than being overweight. I don't take medications. I definitely get my mammogram. I haven't had a colonoscopy yet, but I do all the recommended screening tests. Prior to this conversation, I wouldn't have thought to mention anything about menopause because I wasn't looking at my personal experience of menopause through a medical lens.

Tricia: Yes, yes.

Alexandra: You know I'm fifty-four. My mother died just after she turned sixty, and my father died when he was almost sixty-four. My voice is wobbly as I share that now which reflects that I just don't have the clarity or conviction I would like to have in terms of my health and feeling certain about how much time I have, compared to how much time I want on earth.

Tricia: I want to ask you a little bit more about this because after having taken care of your family for so many years, you're finally in a position to focus much more on yourself. Is that part of this?

Alexandra: It definitely is, but I don't believe it has to be that way. I think it's possible to care for yourself while caring for a family. In fact, I think it's really important to model that for one's children.

It hasn't come easily for me. I've needed to put a lot of deliberate attention into navigating that. I know that's true of many women, but again, I don't think it has to be. We need to learn to honor our experiences more in every phase of life. This isn't only an issue during menopause in the ways we're discussing.

I've created a lot in my life, both personally and professionally. I have given my all to many endeavors and have been gratified with the results. However, I've never really put my attention on my body and my health until recently. My body is an area I've been stuck, and I have been working to change that.

Tricia: Is this all mindset?

Alexandra: Yes, I suppose so, depending on what you mean by mindset. I do think the answer is yes, but not the way most people use the term. "Mindset" often refers to a mental mindset, but when I say yes to your question, I also am referring to the realm of feeling. I think the shift I've described depends on how you feel both about and within your body which is only partially a matter of mental mindset.

I'll say it another way because, for me, so often, things come down to connection and relationship. Previously I've had one kind of relationship with my body, which has included being functional and healthy, present and able to experience a great deal of pleasure, and also somewhat disconnected and overweight. I haven't quite known how to create a different relationship with my body until recently.

Tricia: What does that look like?

Alexandra: Well, I'm going to start my answer by telling you that I rode horses until I was thirteen during summers spent in a rural area and then later while at sleepaway camp. I just loved riding horses.

Tricia: I didn't know this about you.

Alexandra: I had various things happen that ended the horse-riding part of my life for decades.

Tricia: I'm so curious about the "various things".

Alexandra: The first thing that comes to mind is that horseback riding provided a context for a very special connection with my father. When I was a little girl, we'd ride together every summer in the Adirondack Mountains in upstate New York. I'd ride behind my Dad, with my arms around his waist, the way someone would ride behind another person on a motorcycle. I also did a lot of horseback riding at the camp I went to from about ages ten to thirteen. I loved everything about the horseback riding experience. But then, not only did I age out of the camp, but my parents got divorced, and many things changed. One of them was that I no longer rode. This coincides with the onset of puberty for me when I had the experience that my Dad turned away from me.

Tricia: Because he didn't want you to grow up, or something else?

Alexandra: It was complicated. I think, in part, it was because, as I went through puberty, I became more of a reminder to him of my mother and the things he didn't like about her. Another thing is that he dated a number of women after the divorce, but he wasn't honest about it with me. At this point I would say that he was uncomfortable telling me, both because of his own awkwardness discussing his relationships with me and also directly as a consequence of the divorce

In this whole context, there was a time my father promised to take me riding for my birthday. The same year my brother wanted to go to a baseball game for his birthday (which is a week before mine). The baseball game they wanted to go to happened to take place on my actual birthday. I was glad to go to the game, but in the end, we went to the game and never went riding.

Tricia: He didn't just take you on a different day?

Alexandra: No, and I was very hurt. I felt deprioritized in ways I couldn't comprehend. I associate feelings of being so unimportant that he didn't keep his word to me with the end of my childhood riding. In my soul, riding had become intertwined with his broken promise.

Some time ago, my transformational coach said, "What lights you up? What would you love to do, just for yourself, just for the joy of it?" I immediately said, "Horseback riding." Almost a year later, I took action. I found a barn three months ago, and I've been riding every week since. It's the most incredible experience for me, related to my relationship with my body.

The thing I want to say about it is that we are all very familiar with how trauma lives in the body, blocking relaxation, open-heartedness, and new experiences. What I am discovering during my riding lessons is how much joy, connectedness, deliciousness, wisdom, and insight have also been housed in my body. There's so much joy that has been buried in my body in the same way trauma can be buried.

I don't have a childhood home that I go back to. I have hardly anybody in my life who knew me before I was twenty-five years old, which is when I met Rodd. So it has been magnificent to feel these joyful sensations in my body which I haven't felt since I was young. It's a completely different process than accessing what is held in my body as trauma.

I now feel I can connect again to the Dad I had when I was little by taking myself riding. The whole thing is a very profound experience.

I have a lot more joy and connection available in my body that was previously dormant. I have been having great sex, so this isn't about expanding orgasmic experiences per se. It's more about accessing an everyday bounce in my step and having an embodied sense of gratitude. I've realized that for most of my life, I've oriented to my body as a vessel for my soul to live inside of. My body is like the car that my soul gets to drive around in. But I've learned that's not the most attuned relationship I could be having as I am evolving into a more vibrant way.

Tricia: I'm just letting everything you've said wash over me. It's so incredible. We all know horses are such intuitive and divine creatures. I love that you are releasing more trauma and finding more joy.

Alexandra: You know, I don't actually experience it as releasing trauma. For me, it's more like frozen energy melting away. I suppose the fact that it's been frozen does make it sound like trauma. But it doesn't feel that way to me. It's more like there's all this goodness, vitality, playfulness, and harmony that I've been walking around with and not accessing, and now I do.

Tricia: You're making me think again of the time before we moved into this apartment. I didn't realize until this very moment in time that I was carrying the trauma of everyone who lived in that building. Yes, every single person in that building because they all needed my help. I would carry their groceries upstairs. I would teach them how to use the internet. I would call the building superintendent because nobody else would. I was both literally and metaphorically carrying all of their burdens and trauma. Not knowing that, not knowing what that was, but then releasing it, moving here, and then fully tapping into my massive potential has been so pivotal. Yes. Oh, my gosh, I have never framed it like this until just now.

I am certain that this is also part of what set me up to have such a joyous, bountiful, magnificent menopause.

Alexandra: I am so happy for you and glad our conversation allowed that insight to emerge.

Tricia: So much of this is about a willingness to let go so that you are set up for your next phase.

Alexandra: Exactly and when it comes to our bodies, I believe our sensuality can deepen as we age. Whether that happens or not seems to have a great deal to do with whether we take responsibility for our own experiences. Nobody else can provide you with sensuality. It doesn't matter how well your lover touches you; if you aren't embodied, it just won't feel sensual.

Tricia: That's so true.

Alexandra: When I was nineteen, working in southern Germany, I went to a beach in Northern Italy. I saw a group of about twenty men in their thirties. The men were in chairs under colorful umbrellas. Some of the men were fit, and some weren't, but all of them clearly had power. They knew their impact and were used to achieving their goals. I don't know what kind of cars they drove or how wealthy they were, but they had a vibe of moving through life with a lot of power and material success. Nearby there was a group of younger, fit, model-looking women who seemed to be their girlfriends. The women were playing beach volleyball, wearing short shorts and crop tops. They were jumping up and down with their perky breasts and mostly long blonde hair. They really were gorgeous, gorgeous, younger women.

A woman walked along the beach. She was in her late forties or fifties with a rounder physique. She wasn't wildly obese but definitely overweight by American standards. She had cellulite, lots of rolls in her flesh, and she also had much juiciness. She had vitality, self-acceptance, and a kind of wild abandon. She moved down the beach with so much erotic energy. She was glorious!

I watched these men who had these younger, svelte, volleyball-playing, supermodel girlfriends, and I watched as every single one of them turned their heads to watch this woman walk down the beach carrying some packages. Her flesh was magnificently hanging over the top of her bikini bottoms, and all the men were magnetized to her.

Tricia: I can see this happening.

Alexandra: It was a profoundly influential experience for me. As a result, I became clear at a young age that sex appeal and body image are not inherently coupled. Body image and sex appeal influence one another, but a certain type of body doesn't necessarily influence sex appeal. As someone who has rarely been small in my adult life, I deeply appreciated that woman. I loved her without knowing anything about her except what I witnessed on the beach that day.

I've had plenty of thoughts in my head about wanting to have less flesh, but I never was confused that that had anything at all to do with how much pleasure I could have or what my husband and I could experience together with our bodies.

Tricia: So good, so good. I think embodiment is a kind of magic.

chapter 10

SENSUALITY, SEX, AND DESIRE

Tricia: I have always been a sensual creature. I have always asked for what I wanted in the bedroom and in any other room. I think it comes from a place of not knowing any other way—there's been a beautiful naïveté that has served me well. I am not suggesting anyone stay naive, but I think the way I've lived my life, professionally and personally, has always been from a place of making sure I ask for what I want.

Alexandra: How, though? How are you that way? Because you haven't accounted for it in anything you've said. I don't have the impression that it was modeled in your home. I know it wasn't modeled in your conservative midwestern community growing up. Right?

Tricia: None of them. That is one of the questions that many of my mentors are waiting for me to answer. I really don't know. My dance teacher was a huge inspiration for me. She modeled independence. She modeled love. She modeled humor, and she modeled discipline. I guess maybe a lot of this really goes back to her. She ran a dance studio with her mother, two independent women. They were both married to men who were never on the scene. They asked one another for what they wanted. They collaborated with agency and healthy entitlement, and love. I saw that, and somehow, it seeped into me. I took it in and began to emulate it.

Alexandra: And in your childhood home? If it wasn't modeled, were you ever punished or in some way discouraged for speaking up about what you wanted?

Tricia: I remember I was very vocal about wanting to take dance lessons. They were given to me for sure. But then I was punished and shamed for doing homework from 10 PM to 2 AM because I was in dance school until 9 PM almost every day so I needed to do it then. Although it was challenging, it made perfect sense to me. I still got straight A's, so I didn't understand the problem, but somehow my behavior was viewed as abnormal and, therefore, problematic. Being viewed as somehow odd is a longstanding theme in my life.

My intense drive for success, how I have handled myself physically, and my comfort with my sexual expression in relationships and dating is something I have always aligned with. I'm not saying I didn't get my heart broken; I did. But I was always able to have really excellent, pleasurable sex.

Alexandra: From the beginning?

Tricia: Yes. I started having sex with my very first boyfriend when I was sixteen. We were in a monogamous relationship.

Alexandra: Did you talk with your sixteen-year-old boyfriend about sex, or did you just have a naturally curious attitude that resulted in you experiencing a lot of pleasure?

Tricia: Not having a whole lot of confidence or having been taught anything, we fumbled our way through, so yes, I was curious, but not in a mature, "Let's discuss our pleasure" kind of way. We loved each other, so it wasn't casual. Our souls were involved. At sixteen, that can be very dangerous because when that relationship ends, as it should, it is utterly devastating. I didn't know how to break the soul connection when our physical relationship ended. But without that experience, I would not be where I am today, at this moment.

Moving into my twenties, I wasn't available for that to happen again. I wasn't ready, so I wanted my relationships to be simply about fun, enjoyment, and pleasure. Not love.

Then in my late thirties, with Joe, we developed a deep bond of intimacy, love, and commitment. There came a freedom with sex that included conversation. Now, in my fifties, the connection is so strong that when I see him across the street and we're walking toward each other, I get butterflies in my stomach. After thirteen years of marriage, I still get butterflies in my stomach!

When he kisses me in the morning, he does this thing. He puts his arms around me while I'm still in bed and not quite awake, and he kisses me on the lips. With sweet continuous pecks, he says, "I love you, honey, have a good day." That is the kind of intimate bond and sensuality that I'm experiencing now, in my fifties, with my husband.

There's definitely been a true transformation. This is your area of expertise, but I share this for our readers to understand that Joe and I are not having the same sex I was having when I was younger. We are having intentional sex that is extremely pleasurable.

A lot of my friends are dancers, and we laugh because we've all had long dance careers, and now we have to be careful about being on our knees. Sometimes a hamstring will cramp up right in the middle of sex. No joke. Who's talking about that? It should happen more! I do love my body more now than I did when I was sixteen when I was walking around wearing unitards and pointe shoes.

Alexandra: It's so funny to me that you talk about your personal growth journey as having just started five years ago because the way that you talk about the evolution of your relationship is a brilliant example of having a growth-oriented mindset. You had your experience with your sixteen-year-old boyfriend. Then you chose to avoid repeating that dynamic ever again and showed up in the world accordingly. You had that experience, you drew conclusions about it, then you applied them in your next relationships, and you did that more than once. That is being growth-oriented!

Tricia: Yes, and there were lots of times during my twenties when I thought a guy was going to know more than he did. It wasn't good.

Alexandra: You didn't hope it would be better once you got to know one another?

Tricia: Nope. "Next."

Alexandra: Okay, that's remarkable.

Coaching couples on intimacy, there's something that I encounter fairly often; namely, people make assumptions that there's an age that couples stop having sex and uncoupled women of a certain age are no longer interested in sex. Similarly, many people presume they will inevitably run out of new experiences, sexually speaking. Unless in the kink world, people tend to believe a flattening out of passion is inevitable in long-term relationships, as novelty and variety in sex ultimately diminish.

What are your thoughts on this topic?

Tricia: On being married for thirteen years and having sex with the same person? We talk about it. We are both artistic and creative, and we bring that into the bedroom. Also, we plan. Spontaneous sex is very difficult because we are both really busy.

Alexandra: I like how you framed that mature sex includes conversations about it. Talking about sex is everything! Only nine percent of couples who aren't talking about sex with their spouse report being sexually satisfied. In fact, one of the biggest predictors of a long-lasting fulfilling sex life is having conversations with your partner about the sex you're having or want to have.

It's also interesting to keep in mind that you're most likely to have sex again after just having had sex. I don't mean immediately, but the more recently you've had sex, the more likely you are to have it again. The research also says that the thing that makes it most likely you'll have good sex is having previously had good sex. This is a fancy way of saying that our status quo matters when it comes to creating more pleasure. It's almost like a habit that needs to be established.

When it comes to talking with a partner about having better, more gratifying sex, I want to clarify what I am referring to. Discussing anatomy and physiology is important. It's also important to share the stories in your head, how you feel, and how you want to feel. Our primary sex organ is not our genitalia; it's actually our brain. Conversations about sex are one way to use it well to create more pleasure. Other ways to use the brain, beyond fantasy, role play, talking sexy, and that sort of thing, is to use your brain to uplevel your mindset, be intentional about breathing and cultivate attention and presence. Any and all of this leads to extraordinary sex.

Let me emphasize that learning to use your mind well is the best way to resolve many of the issues for menopausal couples, including the big one, namely, thinking that sex is going to be like it was at the age of thirty and if it's not, then it's not worth having.

Here are a few stories to enhance the picture I'm painting. I'll start with a couple I interviewed on my podcast, The Intimate Marriage Podcast. They have been married for fifty-one years. She shared they've always had a solid sex life (with the ups and downs inevitable in such a long marriage). Even so, she's clear she's having the best orgasms of her life now when she's obviously postmenopausal. In the podcast interview, I asked her, "How do you account for that?" She spoke about deliberately enhancing her capacity to experience pleasure and her growing ability to relax into whatever pleasure is available at any given moment. In other words, she is using her mind. The results are spectacular.

I love talking about inspiring couples like this! There's another couple I worked with; they have been married for fifty-three years. She shared they've always had a good sex life, but three or four years ago, they had a "sexual awakening." Now it's even better. It's off the charts! I don't know how old this woman is, but she's old enough to be married for fifty-three years.

These real-life examples are important. They give permission to imagine longevity, aliveness, and enjoyment with conviction. I would also say, from my own experience of being married for twenty-six years and having sex with the same person for twenty-nine, that there's still much variety available to us. It's not necessarily variety in terms of new positions or having sex in new locations or anything so acrobatic. After many decades together, those things are not what create new experiences. I suppose they could, but that's rather uncommon. Variety in the context of a long-lasting relationship is far more accessible in the form of new layers of intimacy and deeper connection.

After decades together, we are more and more attuned to one another's bodies; it makes for much more pleasure. These days, if my husband is inside me and he makes a micro adjustment with his body, suddenly, there's a whole new reservoir of pleasure flooding through my system. If someone happened to be filming our lovemaking for educational purposes, it would not look like anything different was happening. More erotic energy might be perceived, but other than that, it would be as though nothing had happened that was any different than what we've been doing for decades. But the experience in our bodies, well, that's a different story altogether. It's a tsunami of difference, while also one that is nuanced and subtle in its creation.

Tricia: Wow, I find myself going back to the word "capacity." Just look at you. You are fifty-four years old. You are grounded. You're clear. You are very much connected to your body. Your work is growing. Significantly, all of that is true while you are in menopause. I highlight this because everybody talks about a very different version of the menopause experience.

Alexandra: Thank you for that.

Whether I have a new energy and perspective because I'm in menopause, or it's merely that my menopause isn't getting in my way, I definitely feel more vibrant and purposeful than I ever have. For sure, my sex life is more fulfilling than I ever would have imagined it could be when I was a younger woman. It's not that we necessarily have sex all the time. It's a qualitative difference, not a quantitative one. But I do know that if we're going to have sex, it's going to be an extraordinary experience.

Having a nourishing sex life requires conscious attention, putting it in the schedule, and making it a priority. In every other area of life, if I'm not paying attention, I'll be waved down on the highway of my busy life. For example, if I don't pay my bills, I'll get waved down by a reminder notice. If my revenue drops, I'll get waved down. If it rises, I'll get waved down. There is built-in feedback in most areas of life. However, when it comes to our sex life, we continually need to prioritize it because it's very easy for it to slip through our fingers in the busy, full, purpose-driven, meaningful lives we live. When it's neglected, there aren't any external flags that will get our attention or reminder notices that will be sent unless things have gotten very bad.

It's probably worthwhile to name the difference between spontaneous desire and responsive desire here. Are those familiar terms for you?

Tricia: No, but I'm curious.

Alexandra: Spontaneous desire is the kind of desire that is typically felt early in a relationship, if at all. It's the kind of desire that happens when you see your partner and you just want to have sex. In the United States, and probably in many other parts of the world, we think of men as perpetually ready to have sex. That's not actually how I find men to be in my work, but it is definitely the cultural narrative. That assumption is connected with believing most men have spontaneous desire. Responsive desire is the kind of desire that is cultivated; it doesn't arise unless the right things are put in place. For one person that might be needing the bedroom to be cleaned up, candles lit, and a particular scent in the room. For someone else, it might mean particular music, reading erotica, or working out. There are many options, but all of them function to help one get in the mood and to stoke responsive desire. It's very valuable to figure out what you respond to, what turns you on, and what gets your erotic juices flowing. What any given person responds to is going to vary considerably. I believe it's a woman's responsibility to know herself well enough to understand what ignites her desire. Once clear about it, conveying it to her partner is going to be good for both of them. Ultimately, both partners should communicate what they enjoy and what they need to inspire responsive desire.

My husband has learned if he offers me a nonsexual massage, my responsive desire is quite likely to show up. He's very good about how he offers. I don't feel any pressure. I know he's not expecting sex, and I don't feel I am promising it. Through touch, he helps my soul get back into my body. Sometimes after the massage, I'll say, "Goodnight, Sweetheart." But more often than not, I will turn over and be ready to make love.

I'll just repeat that it's a woman's responsibility to figure out what will create responsive desire in her.

Tricia: I love that. What would you say to a woman who doesn't want sex? You've probably coached women who are experiencing painful intercourse, women who don't feel comfortable without clothes on, women who disapprove of their bodies, or any of the many other worries and negative thoughts in our brains that can shut down our bodies.

Alexandra: Yes, I have, and as with any area of personal growth, it's really important to know where you're starting. So if sex is painful, that's important information. If you have body image issues, that's important information. Sometimes a woman doesn't really know what the issue is until she explores it a bit. No matter what it is, the first thing is to put attention to it. That probably sounds obvious, but many women turn their attention elsewhere and need to find the courage and willingness to bring it back to the confronting and complicated matter at hand.

The path to reconnecting sexually is not always about sex or even desire. I'm thinking of a woman I coached who was sexually shut down. Once I understood her situation, I asked her if she had a morning skincare routine. She told me she did. Then I asked her to show me how she washes her face every morning. We were on Zoom at the time. She showed me a disconnected, efficient scrubbing motion. It was the way I would clean a kitchen counter, all practical, without tenderness and care. I invited her to wash her face in a new way, one that was gentler and more loving, which I demonstrated. It was actually confusing to her until I recommended she touch her face the way she had touched her children's skin when they were young. This was her first step in learning to pay attention to sensual experiences. It evolved into guiding herself towards pleasure, first on her own and eventually with her husband.

Tricia: So beautiful.

Alexandra: There are an infinite number of access points to an embodied, sensually rich experience. Each time a woman courageously leans in, it is indeed beautiful. If this were an issue for you (and it's obviously not!), I might start by talking about how you pet your cats, inviting you to notice the kind of caress that feels best to you. Paying attention changes everything. For the most part, it does not take more time to slow down, take a breath, and pay attention during sex.

For that particular woman I was talking about, allowing herself to wash her face in a way that was sensually rich and nourishing was not easy. It was quite confronting. But once she learned how to wash her face in a way that she actually enjoyed, and she had her attention on the enjoyment of it, something big shifted for her. From that moment, she was ready to find her way to stay present and experience pleasure in sex too. This had ripple effects in her choosing what she was going to wear based on the feeling of the fabric that would be touching her skin. Instead of just cooking for health, she learned to cook with the beautiful colors and aromas of the ingredients in mind. She allowed herself to be adequately embodied and present to enjoy her life–all of it. Anyone can experience a similar transformation by slowing down, paying attention, and initially changing the way they do just one thing.

chapter 11

SATISFACTION AND COMPLETION

Tricia: I'd love to go back to the subject of careers because you have said that you feel more empowered now than ever before, especially in the impact you are making in your work. And I want to talk about my career as a dancer too.

Alexandra: Yes, let's.

Tricia: What I'm so excited about is just how much mindset has to do with everything. Most dancers struggle with retiring. I did not. I set myself up very specifically to close that sacred space with intention. I'm not sure I ever shared this with you. I decided to bring my performing career to a close by doing a one-woman show. I had amassed loads of solos from various choreographers over my years dancing with different companies and had started choreographing for myself. I realized I wanted to go out my way.

The process was very much like a sand mandala created by Buddhist Monks. They take much time and care to create it, and once they're finished, they just wipe them away.

I like telling this story. I set up a space for nine months where I rehearsed my solo show. I hired the studio. I booked the theater. I also hired an understudy, so I could see her do the dances.

Alexandra: Oh, my gosh, that's amazing.

Tricia: I hired a dresser too, so in between the pieces, I could rest my muscles. I hired a yoga instructor to warm me up. I started eating in specific ways so that I understood exactly how much energy it would take for me to digest protein versus carbs. There was so much specificity in all of my choices because I wanted to be magnificent. Setting myself up like that has given me the same kind of focus and empowerment for this moment in time. I'm in full acceptance of my body. I'm in full acceptance of the fact that sometimes I actually have to warm up and stretch before sex. That's not a joke. I can't just do a grand jeté.

Alexandra: I don't even know what that is, but I'm going to enjoy imagining it.

Tricia: That makes me smile. I'm reflecting on my current relationship with my body and realizing I love my body even more now than I did while dancing in my one-woman show. I loved her a lot then. Yes, I did. What freedom it is to be fully embodied as a dancer and as a woman, a woman who is fifty-two years old and has zero interest in performing. I am not interested in dancing. I'm not interested in warming up to dance; that part of my life is complete. This feeling of completion is similar to the one you expressed about being complete with childbearing.

Alexandra: I had many thoughts while you were talking. One, which I'll come back to later, is that I think, in our culture, we're not great about transitions, especially transitions of completion. But first, in response to what you said, I want to share that I'm so taken with how fully you gave of yourself in your dance career, which culminated with your show. I believe when you really give all of yourself, it's easier to move on.

The way that I birthed and parented in the early stages of my children's lives, I also feel complete. I don't mean there were no missteps or mistakes. There are a few things I would definitely do differently if I had the opportunity. But I was all in and gave fully, and I think giving wholeheartedly is one of the keys to letting go, of being able to feel complete when the time comes.

Tricia: Yes, that's what we're doing here. I just knew this time with you was going to be a gift. But, my goodness, you have just put it into words so eloquently. For we are giving wholeheartedly here right now.

Alexandra: Well, yes, it's exactly how you did your show. Whether you would have wrapped this language around it or not, that is exactly what you did. Thereafter you could feel complete with your dance career. I believe the feeling of completion is very similar to the feeling of satisfaction. Most women do not allow themselves to feel complete because there is something so vulnerable in satisfaction.

Tricia: Tell me more about that.

Alexandra: Well, most women order short. They don't ask for all of what you want. It's a kind of proactive self-imposed compromise, a bit like not allowing oneself to dream big enough. Both of those modes make satisfaction and gratification impossible because you'll never get everything you want or become all of who you want to be. However, it can feel risky to allow oneself to truly feel satisfied. It requires believing it's possible and then opening up enough to allow oneself to experience it. You have to feel worthy.

Tricia: That makes sense.

Alexandra: You know, listening to you speak about completing your dance career and also your experience of menopause, I'm reminded of how common it is for women to put their joy on hold or make it conditional. They say to themselves, "When I lose fifty pounds, I'll be happy." Or, "When I make six figures, I'll be happy." Or "When I make seven figures, I'll be happy." "I'll be happy when I find a guy." "I'll finally be happy when I have a child." "I'll be happy when I have a boy and a girl." These are all examples of conditions that people believe will guarantee their lasting happiness when it's certainly clear to me that none of those things will do so. It's more important to learn to be happy wherever you are. I hear something equivalent in how you approached these stages of your life. In both instances, your identity conveys how you feel about yourself and who you are, while being detached from needing something in particular to happen in order for you to feel fantastic.

Tricia: I would agree. How I feel about myself in this incredible, beautiful phase of menopause is just wonderful. Menopause, the end of my monthly cycles, has created the beginning of a new generational cycle, a new way of being. It's so different from anything I was taught, and it feels like I'm redefining what menopause can be for myself and for any woman who wants to join me in this invigorating approach to a lifecycle event. This phase feels so fertile, which of course, is wonderfully paradoxical. Consider it: I feel more fertile now than ever before. It's amazing to me that my physiological loss of fertility has given birth to massive creative fertility.

Alexandra: Do you want to say more about that?

Tricia: As I see it, being able to reframe how we participate in our menopause can truly alleviate the suffering that potentially goes on in the process. What are your thoughts?

Alexandra: I teach almost all of my clients how to reflect on the past, how to enjoy reminiscing and sharing insights in a way which allows them to harvest more of the experience itself. Instead of life racing by, we can pause and enjoy what has been without any need to prolong it. Giving it attention allows us to savor it and let it go. Whether it's something big or something more minor, authentically letting it go is very powerful.

Tricia: I can see how it could be fun to acknowledge what happens in your life that way.

Alexandra: Yes, that's so true, whether we're talking about joy, grief, or merely a change in attitude, like reframing our understanding of menopause. It's helpful to look back and connect with how things were while letting one phase go and entering into another. I'm sharing this because I feel a kind of letting go of former attitudes in a way that is actually quite rich, as we each welcome a deeper and far more appealing conception of menopause.

Our cultural narrative around menopause says that it's a time when women become invisible. Looking that squarely in the face this weekend has definitely contributed to my stepping away entirely from that paradigm, both for myself and the older women I interact with.

Tricia: Somehow, this comes back to elegant compensations for me, starting with giving them to ourselves.

Alexandra: Yes, what can make them especially elegant is when we realize our own potency. I am reminded of a study I was exposed to in medical school. It made a huge impression on me, and I think of it often. It was a study done with senior citizens. Each of the participants was put through some memory tests and also assessed for how they walked with respect to pace and posture. Then half of the participants watched a short film in which there were all kinds of images and messaging which conveyed how debilitating aging is. The other group was shown a film that had many positive, inspirational messages about aging. Then both groups were put through the same memory tests and walking assessments. They also measured blood pressure, heart rate, and other physiological parameters at the beginning and after watching these short films. The group that watched a ten-minute film with a depressing message about aging demonstrated a significantly diminished capacity in the memory tests. In addition, they were more likely to be slumped in their chairs, and many of them shuffled instead of walking. The film had an immediate negative impact. Meanwhile, the people who watched the film with positive messaging had the exact opposite results. They walked with upright posture and powerful body language, with no slumping at all. Their memory test scores were higher, and their overall mental alertness improved. What we believe about aging has a tremendous influence on our function. I have been acutely aware of what I tell myself about menopause and aging generally because I know what I tell myself will be extremely impactful. It's a variable entirely independent of any decline in my physiological function.

Tricia: Wow. Do you think it's possible our experiences in menopause feel easier because we started our journey of really clearly identifying who we are and what our purpose, mission, and values are long before menopause began?

Alexandra: Yes, yes, I do. I definitely wasn't that clear about this before we started speaking, but I probably had an unconscious assumption that this was the case. To be honest, I don't know how early I identified my mission. I have done a lot of aligned living, but you seem to have lived your life with a lot more intentionality and focus than I have. I've worked hard and had high standards for myself, but I never identified major milestones that served to propel me forward. For example, I decided to become a physician a year or two before I applied to medical school–it wasn't a path I chose a decade prior and consistently had in mind. I am not someone who was always sure I would get married and have children. I didn't assume I would do either one until it felt right to do so. In contrast, I have the impression that, as far back as you can remember, you have been clear about your goals and precise about what it would take to achieve them.

Tricia: Not necessarily. I mean, I knew I wanted to be different from the older women I saw while I was growing up. I actually remember thinking about that when I was a teenager, but I didn't have any language around intention. I think my growth and evolution consisted of me doing anything and everything I could to avoid repeating the patterns I saw in my life and with my family. But I wasn't conscious of what it means to have a growth mindset until I became conscious through my Buddhist practice. Being proactive and diving headfirst into the power of mindset and intention really only began five years ago.

Alexandra: It's so interesting to hear you reflect on it that way. I believe you, and I feel the truth in what you're saying. At the same time, when I hear your story about being thirteen and knowing you wanted to dance in New York City, it feels different to me. I think of that as having a growth mindset or a growth-oriented trajectory. Maybe it wasn't focused on

SATISFACTION AND COMPLETION

internal truth or inner realities, but it definitely was an example of your ability to imagine yourself accomplishing something in the future and taking action to get there, no matter what was required of you to do so.

Tricia: That's for sure. That is absolutely for sure. Moxie, determination, and discipline all played a massive role. Then later, I learned I was very competent. In fact, because of my drive, I accomplished everything that I wanted and more. But it wasn't until I started really diving into guided meditations and hypnotherapy that I discovered my ability to call in so much more.

Alexandra: That's wonderful to hear.

When you referred to hypnotherapy earlier, I wanted to ask you more about that because it sounds like it's something you do yourself without a practitioner.

Tricia: Correct. I did work with a hypnotherapy coach, Grace Smith. During that time, I received the download that I needed to move. Joe and I had been contently living on 57th Street here in New York for almost fifteen years. When you live in an apartment in New York, and they never raise your rent, you never move. It's very clear. But the apartment was dark. We couldn't grow any plants there. The bedroom faced a bus stop, so we could never open any windows. Then, during the time I was working with this hypnotherapy coach, I got a download. I was preparing for our session, just sitting in the kitchen waiting for her to call me, and I just knew. I thought, "Oh my God, I hope Joe comes with me because I am definitely moving." It was that serious, that clear. When I got that message, I realized that I'd consciously connected to Source for the first time. Knowing that opened up an entire world for me. I realized I can call in a new apartment. Yes, I can. I can call in amazing clients, ones I want to work with in support of my desires. So when I was facing menopause head-on, I realized the same thing applies when it comes to my body and everything else I put my attention on. My inner work got super dialed in. I became conscious. Even though I was competent and successful, I had been unconscious before this happened. It's astonishing how both were true.

I'm grateful I woke up in this way in time for menopause.

Alexandra: I'm glad too!

You know, I very much identify with you. While I didn't have a vision board or definitive life goals guiding my actions, I have definitely been on a growth-oriented trajectory. There's almost always something that I am working on, developing, or cultivating in myself. I've had my moments of insecurity, of course, but in broad strokes, I have been confident in how I have lived. When it comes to parenting, I have trusted myself and followed the beat of my own drum. This has also been true in terms of where we have lived, what kind of food we eat, our children's education, and so much more. I do things my own way in the sense that I am not looking for permission or approval, or validation from anyone else. I've made many significant decisions seemingly spontaneously, without thinking twice. It can feel authentic and uncomplicated, innovative and original, sometimes conventional, but always what's calling to me in a particular instance.

The one area I have not been this way is my business. I have signed up for many different business programs, unconsciously thinking that somebody else has the answers for me. Somebody else has the systems and strategies that will work for me; somebody else has the key. If I just sign up for their program, I'll have it too. That's happened a lot of times. Each one has some value, but none of them has given me the key I was looking for. Indeed I've learned a lot from other people. I'm not diminishing that. And for me, this phase of my life has meant stepping up to the plate and letting go of a childlike identity when it comes to my business. When it comes to coaching my clients, I've always been creative, free, and clear in how I want to serve with depth and efficiency. But with respect to being an entrepreneur, I haven't had that same confidence and clarity.

Tricia: Hmm. Are you now connecting how you are in the rest of your life with your business, learning to show up in similar ways?

Alexandra: Yes, but it took time. I had to evolve to where I now realize that the locus of power is in me, not in any instructor or course I enrolled in. If someone advised me to adopt a strategy, a part of me would believe they knew best what would work for me. Now I pause to consider if I am aligned with it or not, and that's what determines whether I implement it.

Tricia: I notice how quickly you are able to identify when your energy is not aligned with what is being asked of you. That's an important skill.

Alexandra: Yes, I agree. It's one I needed to cultivate. It's actually essential in the work I do facilitating transformation in couples. I am skillful, but it's my alignment that makes me trustworthy.

When I'm doing transformational work with my clients, I take them deeply into my heart. I choose to be fully available while I have my attention on them. I also am clear when it's time to take my attention off them and return to nourishing myself.

Tricia: I love that. And I'm connecting the dots with women who are in menopause. They can go to any doctor they want to and enroll in any program they want to participate in, but it needs to be through the filter of who they really are. Each person's experience of menopause is unique to them, and so they are going to need the support that is right for them.

Alexandra: The word "sovereignty" comes to mind.

Tricia: Yes. So much of the journey we're talking about is individuating and falling in love with who you are and being right with it.

chapter 12

THE IMPACT
OF ENERGY

Tricia: Last night I was telling Joe how I've felt so filled up by our time together. I also told him we would be talking more about sex and energy today. He thought it would be super fun to show you "Sweet Buns."

Alexandra: Great idea.

Tricia: Amazing.

Let me give you some context. I choreographed a piece called "Sweet Buns." It's from a burlesque show, Broadway Varietease, that I directed and choreographed, where I eat a hamburger. (You know I'm a longtime vegetarian, so it was actually a veggie burger). Ready to watch it?

Alexandra: I am. Honored to. Let's do it! [We watched *Sweet Buns*.]

Tricia: I feel so proud to have been able to share that with you. It was a highly choreographed, extremely mathematical dance because I had to literally get a full burger down in three minutes while doing my moves. I knew I could turn my audience on by doing this. But for me, the experience wasn't sensual at all. Think about it. I was focused on the ritual of getting the burger ready, making sure it was the right size, making sure there was enough mayonnaise on the bun so it would slide down my throat, and making sure I had enough cheek room to put it in. It looked like I ate the whole thing. I was performing, and there really was nothing sensual about it for me. But people just loved it. And I loved giving people that pleasure, week after week.

Alexandra: It was so hot to watch! There was no point where you stopped–it just kept going and going, getting more provocative and sexy. Wow. It does feel so good to watch it. I feel I understand you better now. I also feel a deeper level of trust with you after watching it. I wouldn't have expected that.

Tricia: This is so great to hear. Thank you for seeing me.

Alexandra: One of the questions I have for you is this. If you can create so much heat in a calculated performance, how do you make sure your sex isn't performative? Also, knowing now that every move was calculated and that it wasn't a sensual experience for you, it's quite remarkable how much sexual energy was moving through you throughout the performance.

Tricia: There's always sexual energy moving through me. That's something I'm very conscious of and very responsible with.

Alexandra: Yes. You are. I understand how responsible you are with your sexual energy based on how you revealed it on that stage. Simultaneously, you gave a great deal of permission to your audience in terms of their sexual energy. You presented it with pizzazz while also making it very safe.

Tricia: Interesting. Thank you for saying that. You just made me think of something. Many people in the audience later shared with me that they watched my piece and then went home and had great sex. That was always so incredible to hear because, on the surface, I wasn't doing anything except eating a burger, but energetically there was so much more.

Alexandra: So much more!

There's something else, which is integral to our topic of menopause, namely, that our primary way to learn is through imitation. No matter how sophisticated we may feel, humans are still mammals, and mammals learn through imitation. When it comes to our relationships with others, our relationships with our bodies, sex, and communication, and this whole realm, imitation is the primary way we learn. This is why it's such a shame that we hardly have any role models worth emulating. (And anyone who does have a relationship worth emulating tends to be fairly private.)

I used to be extremely private, and now there's very little I wouldn't share. It's not that I want to share the intimate details of my life or that I think people should do things the way Rodd and I do. But I've learned it's quite helpful for people to hear about others' marriages.

I often say, in the context of intimacy coaching with couples, that having a fantastic relationship is a learnable skill. The main reason most people don't have fantastic relationships is a lack of education and role models, and I am doing my part to provide both!

I say all of this because it's clear that the way you danced provided sensual education to your audience. I myself am very inspired, having seen your dance performance and also by what you shared about the rituals you and Joe have. In a way, beyond menopause, this book is also about modeling how to have deep and honest conversations that are nourishing and fruitful.

Tricia: As we were talking earlier about energy being related to visibility, I was thinking about an experience I have every day. I have the pleasure of living in New York City, which means when I'm walking down the street, I get constant feedback that I am visible. Strangers will say, "I love your jacket." Young men will tell me I'm attractive. It's always something. I know it's mainly because of my energy that they see me because this happens when I am out with zero makeup, my hair in a bun, and wearing workout clothes, and I get the exact same feedback as when I'm wearing a gown and fully made up.

I love when it happens. It's not that I need constant feedback, but it's a reminder that feeling invisible probably has more to do with a woman's energy than her age. Perhaps women have allowed themselves to move into a phase where they no longer identify as a woman who has power and sexuality. That would naturally lead to an experience of being invisible. You and I are both very sexual beings. It's just part of who we are. But I also think if a woman wants to, she can reclaim it. That is if she's lost it, or if she's never had it, it can be learned.

Alexandra: I agree. It definitely can. I see it happen in my clients as they wake up aspects of themselves that have been dormant.

There's a famous story about Marilyn Monroe. She was walking in Grand Central Station with a friend of hers. They were just two women having a chat, strolling along, nothing special. In the conversation, the friend made a remark about how it was surprising that the paparazzi were nowhere in sight. Marilyn Monroe turned to her and said, "Oh, you want to see Marilyn?" A change happened instantaneously. It was literally less than a breath. I don't know if she tilted her head for a moment, adjusted her posture, or what exactly she did, but whatever it was, there was a shift. Suddenly there were photographers everywhere, crowds thronging, all wanting her picture and her autograph, yelling questions at her. It was wild. Whereas literally, a nanosecond before, it was just two women walking in Grand Central Station, suddenly a celebrity was present, and the world was responding.

Tricia: Oh my god. I have goosebumps. That's amazing. I've never heard that story before.

Alexandra: A lot of my experience in this phase of my life is about managing my energy and allowing myself to be seen.

I used to have long brunette hair that was thick and beautiful. However, since my hair color changed (first it was salt and pepper, now it's silver), I have received many more compliments than ever before. I had assumed that my silver hair would be noticed less often, but I'm continually proven wrong. In fact, I just had an astounding experience. I'm staying with my friend on the Upper East Side and briefly met her housekeeper yesterday. She immediately said to me, "You're so beautiful, on the inside and out. You're just so special." She said this in such a genuine way. It surprised me. But I get that far more often than I used to when I was younger, with thick brunette hair.

Tricia: Well, I would concur with her about you!

I really do think that the attention we're getting must be, at least in part, energetic.

Alexandra: I totally agree. It's largely energetic. To be clear, I do feel beautiful, and yesterday, I had the kind of glow that comes with having an open heart and feeling fulfilled, which is absolutely how I felt when I left here last night. But it surprised me that someone would see it, put attention on it, and say something lovely to me.

Tricia: I'm curious, what are you intentionally doing to be more visible now so that you can have more impact?

Alexandra: It's mostly mindset. I've been experimenting, and it seems to be working. Here's a funny story about this. I was with a friend of mine, a twenty-eight-year-old woman. We went together to visit friends of hers, a couple. This couple's home is gorgeous, and well appointed. Every room has sculptures, paintings, and gorgeous vases filled with flowers. When we arrived, my friend got into a conversation with the couple. They were fascinated by what she was saying, and none of them were paying any attention to me. It felt strange to me, practically inhospitable. I noticed that I had started to feel small, like a little girl who isn't picked for a sports team during gym class. But then I thought to myself, "Oh, here I am being invisible again." Shortly after, I thought, "This is a choice. Maybe I'm creating it. I'm the one making myself invisible, and I want to stop right now." I didn't want to interrupt their conversation or insert myself into their vibe at the risk of being rude. Instead, without saying a word, I focused on extending my aura. I went from having small, contracted energy to taking up more space with my soul. Does that make any sense?

Anyway, as soon as I extended my aura, they started talking to me. Where I had felt unseen and irrelevant moments earlier, I now felt fascinating and magnetic. It was a very natural, easy, harmonious transition, which led to the four of us having a very dynamic, meaningful conversation in which they asked me lots of questions and leaned in to hear my responses.

Tricia: I relate to that. I've been on stage my whole life, so I've always been visible to audiences. I was the dancer who was very talented but not the most talented. So I had to work harder than others. In adulthood, that served me well, both on and off the stage. However, I soon learned that I could get an audience to do whatever I wanted because of my energy.

I wasn't the most technical of the ballet dancers, but I knew how to pull the audience in. I knew how to take them on a transformational journey from the beginning to the middle to the end, so those in the audience felt like we were all on a journey together, with me leading the way. Being able to tap into who I am, as a performer, and as a dancer doesn't ever go away. I bring it into this phase of my life too.

Being on stage, taking up space, for me, has always been very comfortable. I also understand the responsibility that comes with being this way. You know, I've had relationships with actors and speakers–I don't mean physical relationships, I mean working relationships–where I can see that they are relying too much on what I think. I really want to make sure that they are self-sufficient, and that they are able to take up space too.

What I've come to realize is that facilitating visibility for others is also supporting my ongoing visibility as I get older. We can stay visible, sensual, and powerful, and it takes new forms.

Alexandra: That's such a wonderful perspective.

chapter 13

IN GOOD COMPANY

Tricia: Hello Everyone. Heather, Keiya, Maggie, this is Alexandra.

Alexandra: Hello. Hello. Hello.

Tricia: We are so honored that you are joining us to talk about a really important topic, menopause. Just to give you some context, Alexandra and I spent all day yesterday and several hours today talking about many different aspects of menopause. We are excited to move into the next phase of our conversation and hear from each of you about your own experiences with menopause.

I'd love to start with introductions. If you're comfortable sharing, please talk a little about yourself, how old you are, and what phase of menopause you are in. Heather, would you like to start?

Heather: Hi, I'm forty-eight years old. I'm in what's referred to as perimenopause. I have my period very sporadically. I'll have it, then it goes away for six months, and then it visits me again. So that's where I am in the state of things.

Tricia: Okay. Keiya?

Keiya: Hello, I'm Keiya. I am fifty-five years old. I guess the correct term for where I am is post-menopausal. I live in New York City, and I'm really excited to be here to participate in this conversation.

Tricia: We're so honored to have you.

Maggie: Hey, everyone. I live in the Dallas area. I'm experiencing symptoms of perimenopause too. But apparently, according to my labs, I'm not quite there yet. That part is strange for me. Also, instead of having a lack of menstrual periods, I'm getting periods twice a month. That's not very fun, to put it mildly. I just feel like I'm not myself because, along with these twice-a-month periods, I'm experiencing additional physical symptoms that are getting in the way of feeling like a regular human being.

Tricia: Would you expand on that? Are you saying the lab results don't match up with what you are experiencing?

Maggie: Yes. When my primary provider had my labs drawn, she said, "Okay, even though you're having all these symptoms, you're not in perimenopause." I was concerned and thought, well, what's causing it then? If this isn't perimenopause, it's got to be something else. I decided to seek help from both a chiropractor and an acupuncturist.

My symptoms began with night sweats in my mid to late thirties. I'm a nurse, and I remember the older nurses that I worked with talking about menopause. They would get frustrated when they experienced hot flashes in the middle of the day and complained of sweating profusely at night. I didn't understand what they were talking about until I began experiencing my own symptoms. I remembered those nurses and thought, "Oh, God, what I'm experiencing is probably related to menopause." I never went to get it checked because it was only happening about once a month.

I would also say, in the last five years, my sex drive has decreased significantly. I have no desire. I don't want sex at all. It feels like there is no room for it in my life. I have to mentally prepare myself or, you know, find ways to get myself turned on, to make love with my husband. It was so hard for a while. He took it personally. Obviously, he wanted to feel loved and desired. I do love him, but the physical desire wasn't there. Initially, I thought it was because I'm a busy, driven career mom that I was just focused on other things. But then, more recently, I began experiencing fatigue and brain fog, and weight gain around my midsection. Most nights, I also could not fall asleep. On the nights that I could, I would wake up in the middle of the night and have a hard time going back to sleep. That's when I had all the regular labs drawn. But then I went to a functional medicine doctor. They did a different test called the Dutch test and saw a bunch of different things going on. I also went to an acupuncturist because I just wanted to feel well again.

These days, I don't have any more night sweats. If I do wake up in the middle of the night, I can fall back asleep. I think my energy levels are improving too. My sex drive is back and all of this is because I've been taking supplements and getting acupuncture. Now I'm just focused on the brain fog and the twice-a-month menstrual cycles. But I just feel, "Wow, I wish someone had told me about this or prepared me somehow."

Alexandra: What would you have wanted them to tell you? What would have made this experience less difficult for you?

Maggie: Well, when people talk about their thirties or they talk about getting older, the idea is always that you just have to accept it. But there are ways you can still have a lot of energy and wellness that's the same as in your younger years. I was brought up to believe that because you're getting older, basically, there's nothing you can do about it.

Tricia: That's so interesting, that the labs you had done showed you were not experiencing perimenopause. That's something I find so frustrating. The doctor is saying you shouldn't have a problem because of the lab results, but in reality, you're experiencing lots of symptoms. This was similar to my experience in that one doctor interpreted my labs as saying one thing, and a specialist another, so it was really hard to navigate and figure out what was accurate. I was in uncharted territory and had to find my own way through. That really influenced me and is why we're having these conversations. I want us to be able to learn from one another. It's so important to become aware of our options, compare notes, and support each other.

Alexandra: Maggie, may I ask you two questions?

Firstly, you said you thought your diminished sex drive was related to being a busy career mom and having your attention on a lot of other things. Now that you're taking supplements and getting treatment, your sex drive is back. It sounds like you concluded that it wasn't overwhelm; it was perimenopause. How did you conclude that? What was your thought process? I'm so curious.

Maggie: There was no thought process. It was something I've heard people say. Basically, as you get older, the desire to have sex is going to be less. With me being busy, I literally felt like I couldn't think about it or make time for it anyway.

Alexandra: Thank you. Have you ever discussed menopause with your mother?

Maggie: No, that's definitely not something that she would ever be open to talking about.

Tricia: Thank you for sharing so vulnerably, Maggie.

Alexandra: Yes, I think your voice represents so many women. Thank you for your honesty and transparency.

Tricia: Keiya, would you like to tell your story next? Of course, this can be an open dialogue and more popcorn-style as well.

Keiya: Sure, I'm glad to tell my story. I mean, Maggie just pretty much nailed my experience. One thing that was a little different for me was that I did not have hot flashes. I think my menopausal journey started probably around the time I turned fifty. That would be five years ago. I had no hot flashes. So I was happy, feeling like I was beating this thing. I was excited because all the stuff that I'd heard about menopause wasn't happening to me. I also was in a unique situation because I was a flight attendant. I was constantly on the go, traveling back and forth to Europe. So the fatigue I was experiencing, it was easy to assume it was just part of flying. I thought I just couldn't catch up on my sleep.

I think it started hitting me that something else was going on when the lack of sex drive got really strong. But then I thought again, well, fatigue and flying, that explains it. But what made it really challenging was the vaginal dryness. So even when we actually tried to have sex, it was so painful for me. I had no idea what was wrong. At that point, I hadn't even read about menopause. It wasn't until COVID happened, and I took time off from work, and I had to slow down, that I realized a few things. I'm not on the plane. I'm not flying. I'm on leave. I'm not doing all the things that contributed to all of the stuff I was experiencing, but I'm still feeling the same. Actually, I'm feeling worse. That's when the brain fog really came in, as well as mood swings too. I still never had the hot flashes, but then, much like Maggie, I just knew something was wrong.

At this point, I went to multiple doctors, and they did bloodwork. I even went to a gynecologist and an endocrinologist. With each one, I continued to hear, "Everything is fine," or "You're fine. You're really fine." There was a little bit of, "Well, you know, this hormone is in the low range of normal, but it's still in the normal range, so don't worry." But I just knew something was wrong. I decided to try taking various supplements though I wasn't really experiencing any major changes. This went on for a year.

It wasn't until I was actually working with a client and I just could not concentrate. Mentally nothing was happening. I was on a Zoom call with her and I was a mess. She said, "I know what's wrong with you. You need to get in touch with my hormone doctor right now." So that was the changing point for me. When I went to the hormone doctor, I had bloodwork done and she was the first person to say to me, "How are you functioning? You have no testosterone. You have no hormones." I felt so validated and also hopeful because, finally, someone was telling me what was going on.

All those things that happen in menopause, in terms of your hormones, got worse during that time. Also, I had spent such a long time not realizing that something was actually wrong, meanwhile attributing it to something else. Anyway, I remember being really angry. I was really fucking pissed off. What really annoyed me, and pardon my French, but I was just outraged, was this. First of all, I'm going to all these doctors, and I'm saying something is wrong with me. They just tell me, "Oh, yeah, blah blah blah, we'll try this. If that doesn't work, we'll try that." I got the feeling, similar to what has already been shared, that they were saying that what I was experiencing was normal. It completely undermined my concerns. It was kind of like, "Ok, you're menopausal." I took that to mean they considered it normal to have an unfulfilling life. It was considered normal to be fatigued, miserable, have no sex life, and all because I was going through menopause! That is what really annoyed me. It felt like I was being told that I was doomed and there was nothing to do about it.

That's when I felt I needed to start researching for myself. I started speaking to people, and they would say, "Oh, yeah, that's how this goes." I would think to myself, "Well, how come no one ever said anything to me about this? Why is this brand new information?" From then on, I made it a point to start speaking to people in my life about this. They responded by saying, "Oh my god, I'm feeling this way too." I definitely make it a point to share this. I'm not going to let other people go through the shit I went through just because no one talked about it. It was incredibly hard, devastating, actually.

My route out of this mess has been bioidentical hormone replacement. I started taking them a year ago, and it's been life-changing. However, I did have some complications initially, but I think it had to do with the practitioner more than anything else. I've gone on to work with someone else, and everything is improving. At this point, I'm still dealing with some fatigue; however, I've recently found a new holistic doctor to address that. I also have brain fog still, but my sex drive is definitely back, so I'm very happy about that. There's no more vaginal dryness, which is good! I remember the first time we did it after a long time. I felt so glad we didn't have to struggle and fight about it anymore.

Tricia: That's a lot. Thank you for sharing, Keiya. I really want to highlight that both you and Maggie were completely dismissed by your first doctors. I'm sure there is a connection between women feeling invisible as they age and being dismissed by their doctors and others in positions of authority. I'm just highlighting that as part of the story that we're telling in this book; the external world is not supporting, and maintaining, women's visibility based on how many healthcare providers are not showing up for us.

Alexandra: Keiya, thank you. There's something about your experience of menopause, and Maggie's, that makes me think of girls who are never told anything about menstruation. When they begin bleeding, they think they are dying because they have no context to understand what is actually going on. It's obviously not literally equivalent, but there's a way in which both of you were incredulous that no one told you anything about what you might experience in menopause. In both cases, it seems like an analogous, irresponsible lack of education. I would also love to ask you, before we move forward if one of you could offer some specificity to describe your experience of brain fog?

Keiya: Sure. Ordinarily, I'm pretty focused. If I put my mind to something, I do it. There's no question. It's so funny because I was working with Tricia at the time my symptoms were escalating. I remember thinking, "This woman must think I'm a complete loser because I just wasn't able to follow through on anything." Integrity is really important to me. My word means a lot to me. If I say I'm going to do something, I will do it. During that time, I found I just couldn't think straight. Suddenly, I had a profound lack of focus. I would read something and immediately forget it. I'd have to go back and read it again, though I would probably forget again. I had so much brain fog, and before menopause, I never had any of these problems. I'd have momentary little spurts where I would be okay, but then it would come back, and I'd say, "Oh, God, help me. I can't even think right now." Thinking was painful.

Tricia: Was there any sense of relief when you learned this was directly related to hormone imbalances rather than character and it could be corrected?

Keiya: Oh, yes, that was a huge relief. For me, not being able to honor my word to myself and to others was not acceptable. If I had not found a solution or an answer to that, it would have done me in. It really would have. So it was a massive relief for me. I felt grateful, saying, "Oh, thank you, God! I'm not crazy. I'm not losing my mind. I'm not suffering from depression again. Thank you." I know some of you don't know my story, but I have suffered from depression, and I survived a suicide attempt. So for me particularly, all of these menopause symptoms were extra scary. I couldn't handle depression coming back. I just couldn't go down that path again, so yes, it was a huge relief.

Tricia: Thank you for sharing so eloquently.

Keiya: Alright, you tell me if it's too much.

Tricia: I want all of it.

Alexandra: I do too.

Keiya: Thank you.

Tricia: Heather, would you like to share?

Heather: Sure. I can relate to a lot of what's been said so far. In my twenties and thirties, I was a professional dancer. I retired from the dance world around forty and began teaching fitness, working on my own business. My weight started to creep up. I was super aware of it despite no changes in my diet or fitness routines. That was the first thing that got my attention. This is not okay. This is not fair. I exercise. I don't overeat. I have a drink every now and then. I don't smoke. Why is this happening to me?

I didn't put much thought into it because I was busy trying to build my company. Then boom, I started to get my period so severely, at least two times a month for eleven days at a time. I was incapacitated, but I still had to get up at 4 AM and teach at 6 AM. I thought, "Oh my goodness, I am paying for getting my period so late in life." I did not get my period until I was seventeen and only had one cycle. I didn't get it again until I was eighteen. Because I'm a dancer, it was very irregular for my whole twenties. So I was thinking, "This is payback. I am now having double periods for all the years I missed." I had all that going on, and then I knew I was starting to experience depression. I couldn't quite put my finger on the term, but I definitely had tipped into a place where I wasn't happy with anything or anyone, including myself. It was really difficult. That's when we were hit with the pandemic, so I postponed my gynecology visit.

Before all this happened, I liked her because she never pestered me about my decision not to have children. Anyway, I eventually went in for an appointment. I explained everything, and she was very dismissive of my concerns about my weight gain. She said, "Well, it happens." No, it doesn't happen! I'm doing all the right things, What's going on? Not once did she mention menopause. So then I told her how badly I was bleeding. She recommended a transverse ultrasound. It also seemed like she couldn't keep my story straight. After I had the ultrasound and other tests, I really felt brushed off. The pandemic was in full swing, so no one was seeing patients in person. At this time, she called me and said, "Well, we don't really see anything much except for a very thin lining of your uterus." She informed me she was going to take me off the pill. As somebody who's been on the pill for my whole adult life, I didn't think about what would happen when I went off it. I didn't anticipate suddenly being without those hormones anymore. She certainly didn't say anything about it. Pretty quickly, I realized that the birth control pills had been helping to keep me afloat. Her idea was that going off the pill might stop the heavy periods. Well, not only did going off the pill stop my period, I went six months without getting one.

I went into a deep depression. I had to get antidepressants because I was falling off the cliff. I actually dropped weight at first, probably because of stress. It was rough. Then came the vaginal dryness; that was something I had never experienced before. It stopped my drive completely. I didn't even realize how much I had taken normal daily wetness for granted until it went away completely. I felt uncomfortable just sitting, like uncomfortably dry. I was plummeting. So I went to a doctor to do a blood test, and a full workup. She says, "Well, we're reading the numbers, and it looks like you're in full-blown menopause." Now the problem is that when they take your blood work at that moment, they don't consider ranges. You're either pregnant or you're in menopause, The numbers are the same regardless of what is causing the hormonal changes. She says, "You're obviously not pregnant. So you may possibly be in full menopause. How many months have you missed?" It had been six at that point. By the time I was tested again, because I'd been doing blood work every six months, the results showed I was in perimenopause.

I ended up going to see a different gynecologist, and finally, after six months, I got my period. This is when I learned I could become aware of when I was ovulating and when I was going to get my period because ovulation is one of the only times I get a little wet. I still go months without having a period. But when I do get it, the period is really, really bad. Anyway, I went to a new gynecologist who did another transverse ultrasound. She tells me, "This is very common in perimenopausal women. You have a huge fibroid embedded into your uterus wall. No wonder you're bleeding like this." Then, she went back and looked at my old test and saw the first gynecologist had brushed over it. But it was there. It was hard to hear that it was noticeable the first time, but nothing was done about it. I just heard, "Well, let's take you off the pill, or let's wait and see." No one took me aside and said, "I don't care, pandemic or not; you need help." That's where I am in all of this.

I do feel my depression has gotten a little bit better. I always feel better mentally when I get my period. Then I plummet when my hormones plummet. That part is still very scary for me. I just got my period last week after not having one for five and a half months.

My other main concern that I'd like to bring up is women like me who are not having children. I've been told by doctors that we are at a higher risk, especially with small breasts and dense breast tissue, and not having children. We're at a higher risk of getting breast cancer and uterine cancer. If you take prolonged hormone replacement therapy, you are also put in a high-risk category for breast cancer and uterine cancer. So for someone who is already highly susceptible to getting these cancers, and then taking hormone replacement therapy long term, it puts me at an even higher risk for cancer. Where are the better options? Why aren't there solutions that could work for me?

I also went to see a holistic practitioner that was not covered by my insurance while I'm already oozing out money to my insurance company. I noticed none of the things that seemed like they might help are covered. I hope your book includes these things because they really matter.

Tricia: I love you so much. I'm so emotional now. You've shared this with me before, but sharing it like this in an open forum is powerful and important. I can see your pain, and I empathize with your struggle. I can see how hard this is and that you have not been given the support you need, the support we all need and deserve. We have to change that! We need to have these kinds of open dialogues.

Alexandra and I are both having our own experiences of menopause. Our experiences are quite different from the three of yours. I say that because I want to give voice to the fact that there is no "one size fits all" when it comes to a woman's transition out of fertility, out of girlhood, into new possibilities, which are at once both exciting and challenging. I'm hoping that this conversation will inspire many more conversations, especially among women, but also among families and health care providers. Alexandra, do you want to chime in?

Alexandra: Yes, I want to acknowledge each of your individual experiences and your suffering too. I have to add, on a personal note, that I don't practice clinical medicine anymore, but I'm connected with women physicians around the world. What the three of you just shared is very much the result of a male-oriented, male-developed medical system, which obviously can negatively affect individual women's experiences with their individual health practitioners. Not that long ago, all medical research was only done on men. It was only in 1993 that a federal law was passed requiring that women and minorities be represented in the funding of clinical trials. That's when the law was passed, so you can imagine that it takes years for the first studies to be funded and many more years for useful data to be collected and available for clinicians. Prior to that, women's bodies were viewed as too complicated, with too many variables that couldn't be controlled. This means more than half the population wasn't having relevant research done, so how are doctors going to have treatments available and learn how to provide medical care for us. I believe this had and continues to have very real consequences simply because doctors don't have adequate information or training.

As a result, there is a widespread phenomenon, which all three of you exemplify, where women are often caught between scientific, research-based, insurance-covered care, which is inadequate, and alternative, holistic care for those who can afford it. I want to strongly recommend the North American Menopause Society. The website is www.menopause.org. The society provides evidence-based, compassionate training for doctors and others who treat patients in menopause. You can use the site to look for a practitioner where you live. If you're going to pick someone from a list of random doctors covered by your insurance, look for someone who is NAMS trained and certified.

Heather: I'll definitely look into it.

What's so crazy about all of this, and really makes me mad, is that every single woman on this planet will go through this, every single woman! If a man can't get his dick up, there's a pill to fix the problem. Right? Not every man is going to experience a need for Viagra, but it's available to him in case he needs it. Yet every woman is going to go through a big life-changing thing without adequate medical support. It's ridiculous and so sad too.

Tricia: Can I share an observation, Heather? It's something I want to highlight, namely, that all three of you are deeply connected to your bodies. I've known Heather for a really long time from our work together in the theater. Heather is, and will continue to be, my muse forever as far as choreography goes. Heather, you have been so in touch with and in control of your body for decades–whether it's how high your leg goes or how flexible you are–I can see how being so out of control has been devastating for you. I acknowledge that.

Heather: Thank you.

Alexandra: It also sounds like all three of you have been in an argument with your body. Each of you has used different words to express it, but you all describe not feeling on the same team as your own body, feeling like you can't trust it to behave as you want and need.

Tricia: Would you like to expand on what it means to not be on the same team as your body?

Heather: I think it's a war that I've been in my whole life. It's actually very hard to separate it from menopause and everything else. I always needed to be a certain size, or at least attempted to be, for my whole career. The lack of control I felt to even be able to achieve it! I've had this war going on my entire life. It's really hard to separate it out, but I do know that this time it's a totally different game.

Alexandra: How is perimenopause different from the ongoing war?

Heather: Well, before all this, I felt I could control things. I just would eat a little less of this or that. Overall, I would lose weight. Whereas now it sits on my hips and my belly. It doesn't matter if I eat fewer calories. Eating less actually seems to damn me even more. I've tried eating more protein, but I'm a muscular person, so when I up my protein, I get even bigger and bulkier, not leaner. It feels like this process is making everything even more unhealthy in regard to my relationship with food. It's not that I don't eat; it's just an unhealthy obsession constantly. Also, because I now teach fitness, people look at me and judge; well, if you teach fitness, you should look like a twenty-year-old or somebody on Tiktok or some other platform. You should look like those kinds of people, right? I'm thinking, no, they spend six hundred and ten hours a day working out. I teach people how to work out. So it's different.

I don't know if I can elaborate much more on the difference between my ongoing struggle and how it's been recently.

Tricia: You did it beautifully, Heather.

Maggie, what about you and your relationship with your body?

Maggie: I echo everything Heather just shared. I think there's a lot of weight shaming, not just in America but in every culture. I'm sure there are cultures where being full-bodied and curvaceous is a beautiful thing. But culturally, at least in the Vietnamese culture that I've grown up in, they will tell you very directly that you need to go work out. Sometimes that's the first thing that comes out of their mouths. "Oh, you got really fat. You need to go work out." Maintaining a body that I feel good about has always been something that I have tried to control.

In high school, I was bulimic. It wasn't until I started nursing school and truly understood my body that I realized that's what my behavior was. I knew I was hurting my body with what I was doing, but it was more important for me to look good. I've recovered from bulimia, but I think parts of that mentality and conditioning still live in me. I definitely notice if I can't fit into the jeans that I really like. I've really struggled trying to figure out what works for my body. I can't do high cardio type workouts because my body holds on to that weight. But mentally, I feel like I can't lose weight unless I sweat my ass off. So there's always a struggle to find what works well for my body in terms of maintaining my weight, feeling healthy, and being happy with the way I look, even if I'm not the same size or shape that I was in my twenties.

Honestly, I don't feel like I'm forty-six, though I am. I still feel like I'm in my twenties. That's a battle I'm in. I'm forty-six, but I don't feel like I'm forty-six. That's why I keep fighting because I don't have to be so uncomfortable and live this way. I know I can feel better. I know I can live better. Because what would feeling forty-six be like? It would feel like what my friends feel like when they complain about achy joints and other problems. I mean, why care about being tired when they are complaining about exhaustion? I associate that kind of exhaustion with what forty-six would feel like to me. And I definitely refuse to be like that. I believe we are in control. We have control of our bodies. We have control over how well they function, and there are ways for us to change things. We don't have to settle. There's no more just accepting that we have to age and suffer through things.

Alexandra: Might you consider that feeling like forty-six includes feeling great? I'm wondering if feeling great is necessarily only associated with being in your twenties?

Maggie: Right. I guess I would consider that. When I feel great, I will consider that forty-six can feel great.

But right now, it's hard because I want something, but my body is behaving differently. It feels another way. And the people around me who are my age or older, very few of them feel amazing, awesome, and healthy. They don't have vitality.

Alexandra: Well, I definitely feel that way. I'm fifty-four. I'm overweight. I haven't ever had the body that you all describe as having had in your twenties and thirties, so I don't have a sense of having lost my physique in the way you do. I would have liked to have that kind of body, but I never did.

Tricia: Yes, and if you consider how many different versions of the menopause experiences there are in the world, that provides perspective too.

Multiple times this weekend, Alexandra and I have used the word "sisterhood" as we continue to imagine a collective sisterhood engaging in open, honest dialogue. Because how many of us have felt alone or crazy? How many of us have experienced catastrophic thinking? I notice when I'm moving through any kind of transition into my next natural alignment, I truly don't know how long it's going to take until it's completed. So what the fuck do we do while we're here, while everything is out of alignment, including our hormones and the havoc that wreaks? In my opinion, this conversation is part of the treatment.

Keiya: I'll share about my body too. To start with, my nickname growing up was Sexy. I always thought I was sexy, and I've always loved my body. It wasn't until I started going through menopause that I realized I was gaining a little weight, and, unlike every other time, I wasn't able to lose it. I had always maintained a certain weight of about 115 pounds. I was fifty when my weight crept up. But for me, I think the bigger issue was that my vitality was missing. The journey I've been on happened in a way that required me to feel acceptance. It's part of how I've processed it all. I am currently doing things to get my vitality back, such as taking bioidentical hormones.

Where I'm at now is accepting my body without the vitality it had before. But also, at the same time, being in a place of thinking about what I can create from where I'm at with the energy levels I currently have. I'm also focused on looking at things from the perspective of me being fifty-five, my body looking the way it does, and really giving myself more positive feedback about my body. I make a point of saying to myself, "Oh my god, I looked so good. I looked so hot." As a matter of fact, when I was getting dressed today, I thought, well, it doesn't really matter how I look cause they're just using the audio. And then I thought, "Yeah, but you know, I want to look good because I want to feel sexy." I really feel I've been on a journey where I've fallen in love with my body again. I used to have a hard body, but that's no longer available to me. I've tried everything I can to lose the extra flesh, but now I say, "Okay! I'm good with this." That's my journey with my body, and I feel really good about where I'm at.

Tricia: I love hearing this notion of acceptance with grace. It's powerful. I think there is a very important difference between resignation and acceptance. I also feel that our relationship with our bodies and the weight we are right now is not necessarily directly related to menopause. It's something that Maggie referred to earlier. Culturally, we're all obsessed with the scale. At least we are in this country. But something you also talked about, which is so important, is that when I look at my body without clothes on now, I notice my skin is different. But I'm grateful that I still have skin, that I'm clearly alive. With that awareness, I can live in my body even if it's not as supple as it once was.

Alexandra: Yes, absolutely.

Tricia: My boobs are not as high up on my ribcage as they once were. Cellulite has appeared in new areas. Hair has started growing more on my chin and less on my head. All these things happen, they happen. That's just the way it is. For so long, at least in the way I experience the culture, there have been such negative connotations about all these things from all spheres. Even Nora Ephron, whom I definitely consider a feminist, wrote something about always needing to wear a scarf and never letting anyone see her neck ever again once she'd noticed that her neck looked older. But see, I don't plan on making myself small for anyone, creepy neck or not.

I will not stop wearing a swimsuit when I'm in Mexico with my husband, just because I'm fifty-two. I refuse to make myself small. I refuse to give up my sexuality or my sensuality. Why should I? I'm not saying that hormonal changes, and everything that comes with them, are not challenging or things to contend with. But I also think menopause is often treated as yet another negative cultural message, broadcasting to women that they need to hide away and become invisible. And if medical professionals we trust say, "Sorry, the labs aren't telling us anything. So there's no problem." Well, to that, I say, "There is. We are, we are your problem, and we need quality healthcare."

Our lives and experiences are meaningful at every age. Until we have open dialogue, until we have authentic conversations, like the one we're having now, about all the variations in how women experience menopause, women are going to keep disappearing. They're going to keep listening to their doctors belittling their concerns and experiences, and that is not okay!

Alexandra: Each of you is so articulate and generous in sharing your experiences about the changes you've noticed in your bodies and in your emotional landscapes. I would also love to hear from each of you about your relationships with significant others or anyone else in your life, such as your parents, friends, and coworkers. What has the impact been? What have you noticed?

Maggie: I don't know how much my relationship with my two teenage boys is influenced by where I am in my life versus their behavior because it's such a complex interaction with them. Sometimes I think it's just that I am much more easily irritated—much, much more.

Alexandra: May I ask you about that? There's feeling more easily irritated, more easily annoyed at things. And then there's the feeling, "I'm just as irritated as before, but I'm not putting up with things as much as I used to." It may look the same to your family, but I'm wondering if you feel you're really more irritated or that you've always been that irritated, but you put a lid on your reaction prior to this phase of your life?

Maggie: I think I'm really just more irritated. I'm also more reactive than I used to be. I will say, now that you've brought it up, that I probably do express it more too. Through this process, the most significant relationship that has been affected has been the one with my husband. That's from the lack of intimacy related to my diminished sex drive. Otherwise, he's very patient with me. He's compassionate when it comes to my moments of irritation and reactivity. But the side to our marriage, where we are expressing our love for each other, is different. When that was lacking, that was really hard. While it was happening, I couldn't explain it in any other way except to say that I was busy. I mean, that's actually what I really thought it was, and I truly was busy. I couldn't fit anything else into my head or into my life. Trying to force sex was difficult because you can't force that. You have to want it.

I'm actually doing the testosterone pellets now. I didn't do much research before starting because I was so desperate. I'm happy and satisfied that they work, and it's definitely improved our relationship because it gave me the solution to why I was feeling that way. In any case, I would say that the relationship in my life that was most affected was with my husband, which it turns out was all due to me having low testosterone levels. I think just being unhappy is probably what's triggering everything else.

Tricia: May ask you a question?

Maggie: Yes.

Tricia: Will you be talking to your sons about sex?

Maggie: Oh, we already have.

Tricia: Have you ever considered up until this moment in time having a talk with them about menopause?

Maggie: No. I've never considered it. But I will say that I'm sharing a little bit more openly about how I am feeling at this age and how I feel about aging. I don't want them to also feel like giving up when they don't feel well because they're maybe in their fifties or sixties. What was that word you guys used? "Resignation." Right? That's how my husband was. He's in his early fifties now, and he's pretty much given up. He says, "Well, it's just a part of aging." I keep saying, "No, you are not an old man yet." So having that conversation with my sons? Yes. But I would not have considered the menopause discussion with them.

Tricia: I bring it up because Alexandra and I talked about elegant compensation. What I mean by that is learning to make accommodations with kindness and respect. For example, in the apartment I share with my husband, the air conditioner is often on. Rather than discussing the temperature, or shaming me, or saying something along the lines of "I can't believe it's so cold in here," Joe, my husband, simply puts on a sweater. He loves me, he understands this time in my life, and he simply puts on a sweater. I'm sure his mother did not teach him about menopause, but he's certainly a very well-educated husband when it comes to menopause and my relationship with it. I never really thought about how that happened for him, either.

Maggie: I definitely think it wouldn't hurt to have that discussion if my sons are open to hearing it. Although I think it would be more about weaving it into regular conversations rather than a whole formal sit-down event. It's not like the sex conversation where they need specific information in order to proceed with their lives in the near future. It's more about normalizing this topic in a way that I'm guessing none of us experienced in childhood.

Alexandra: Heather, would you like to talk further about your relationships?

Heather: I can say something. To start with, I didn't have a very open conversation with my mother about any of this.

Definitely not. I also just had a uterine cancer scare that prompted me to start asking her questions about menopause, but she had a hysterectomy. She couldn't remember what year she had it. She couldn't remember anything, let alone how it sent her into early menopause. I also wanted to know when it happened because my period stopped for months at a time at age forty-five. That's considered early, so I wanted to know how it was for her, but I couldn't even get timelines from her to help me know what to expect. But the truth is, I don't think she would discuss it openly anyway, even if she and I were better at communicating.

I definitely know that I struggle with things like the air conditioner, and there is a lack of compassion about it towards me. It can almost be a downright drag-out fight about it. It's especially hard for me because my partner went through all this with his ex-wife. But my journey through it is completely different from hers. So when someone says to me, "I understand what you're going through. I went through it." With my husband, I'm like, "No, you don't understand anything. One, you didn't go through it. And two, I'm not having anything like the experience you assume I'm having." As we've said, there's a different journey for each person.

Tricia: Do you feel alone in your experience of menopause?

Heather: Definitely. I don't talk about it very much. I compartmentalize it. Also, I think the pandemic amplified it, kind of pushing me to focus on it. I was busy, still working, but in a different sense because I was at home. I was stuck at home, then taken off the pill, and went through everything that followed. So definitely, yeah, I feel like I've been very alone on this journey.

Alexandra: If you were able to influence your partner, and you wanted him to understand one truth about your situation, what would you want him to know?

Heather: I would want him to know that I feel completely helpless sometimes, and it feels completely out of my control. I actually really need compassion. I want a gentle hand. I said this earlier, but I'll say it again. I need it easy right now; I truly need that. Sure, that's going to be very hard for some people to wrap their minds around, especially when they haven't experienced it. I've learned that some people really need to experience something themselves in order to understand it. So yeah, the truth is that what I want most is compassion.

Alexandra: Thank you, I get it. I feel like you're saying if you broke your leg, it would be more convenient because your husband would understand it more. Likely you would experience more compassion without any need to explain or defend yourself.

Heather: Yes.

Alexandra: Thank you. Thank you, Heather.

Keiya: I guess it's my turn. It's interesting because I'm always cold. I had no night sweats and no hot flashes. So I have the complete opposite experience in that regard. Anyway, in terms of relationships, I am really blessed and fortunate. My husband has always been very, very understanding, even in terms of vaginal dryness, and going through the whole journey with me when I was looking for doctors and all of that. I think even when we initially started having sex, when it became a challenge, he was always very understanding and nurturing. Going through the whole journey, he's been very supportive.

I never had a conversation about menopause with my mother, who is no longer here. In my culture, West Indian culture, that conversation is not going to happen because they don't think you should have sex until you're one hundred years old!

One place I feel menopause actually helped me was in my relationship with myself. It required me to slow down more and really take care of myself. I started to notice and respond to my needs because I couldn't bypass them any longer. I'm a doer. I like to keep going. During this time, it was oh, no, no, no—I couldn't do things even when I wanted to. So I connected more with myself and what I needed to take care of myself. It was really beneficial.

My relationship with my colleagues and business suffered because I needed whatever energy and vitality I had to take care of myself. Additionally, with the brain fog, it was hard to follow through on things. I just couldn't do it. I suffered quite a bit from this, but I think now there's a benefit because it's helped me become more alert to other women when they're sharing things with me. As I've mentioned already, if I suspect another woman might be going through the same thing that I'm going through, and they have no clue what's going on, I become a good resource for them. That's how it's played out for me.

Alexandra: That's beautiful. When it comes to colleagues and business, do you also see an impact in terms of some amount of revenue opportunity lost? Or is it more subtle?

Keiya: Yes, I do, in the sense of needing to turn down opportunities that probably would have led to an increase in revenue. I declined certain opportunities because I felt I couldn't do the work. I would never want to say yes, and then not be able to follow through. This all happened during the time I was playing around with writing my own book. That occurred in the height of all of it, but it just couldn't even happen. I couldn't exert the effort necessary to write a book.

Tricia: Spending time constantly going to doctors must have impacted your revenue stream as well. Is that right?

Keiya: I would say yes, that definitely impacted my finances because my insurance covers almost nothing, and it's all incredibly expensive. My deductible is $7,500. For a person paying for an individual plan that covers basically nothing until the deductible is met, and then suddenly I had to have another ultrasound, and a hydro sonogram too, and this and then that. It all adds up, but I had to have all these extra things as part of getting to where I could feel better. So I was paying huge amounts of money, all out of pocket, during the entire two years of COVID, which were anyway financially stressful. My insurance never paid for anything. Insurance companies, our whole present healthcare system, don't really help with menopause symptoms. Maybe I'm getting off track—I'm not sure if this is relevant.

Alexandra: I think what you are saying is incredibly relevant. Good care and treatment for women in menopause should not be a privilege; it should be a right.

Keiya: Yes, it's extremely important. My relationship has suffered, too, because when I come home, I've already depleted all forms of positivity with my clients. I literally give it to them all day. So by the time I come home, the depression is heavier. I'm exhausted, and all of those things that go with it. I feel rage all the time and such anger.

Alexandra: I'm curious if you know what exactly you're angry about? Is there an object of your rage, or is it not directed at anything in particular?

Keiya: I would say there are a couple of things. I'm angry at the dismissal from doctors in particular. They behave as if it's normal to be miserable. I'm angry at insurance companies. As I mentioned before, they do not cover anything. I believe insurance usually covers Viagra. But when it comes to supporting women as they go through menopause, with whatever treatments or support they want or need, insurance doesn't cover most of it. It has to be paid out of pocket. There's quite a lot to be angry about, but those are two of the biggest things.

Maggie: I have to think about what I'm angry at. There are so many things that go on during the day, and I'm just so snappy. Dismissal is definitely something that triggers me, with my kids too, when they don't hear what I'm trying to say. Sometimes they just walk away while I'm speaking. Dismissal with anybody is infuriating, but I think it bothers me with my kids most of all because I love them, and we have such a close relationship. In terms of other people, it's hard to say because my reactivity and irritation are probably directed more toward my family than anyone else.

Tricia: There's something I want to observe. It's that fighting for your health or fighting for your recalibration seems to be a full-time job. It makes sense to me that so many women just give up and become invisible. The energy it takes to fight for your health, especially the high level of health that you want and know is possible. It's just so exhausting and demeaning. I now understand why so many women in menopause become deflated, dehydrated, and small. I'm so grateful that each of you agreed to have this conversation with us. It's incredibly enlightening for me, a woman who is in menopause herself, to hear about your experiences.

Alexandra: Do you want to say anything about your rage, Heather? Or do you feel complete?

Heather: Are you asking about what enrages me daily or about my feelings toward menopause in general?

Alexandra: Really, I'm glad for you to take it however you want to. I'm familiar with generally walking around in a cloud of rage. And then there's having rage towards something or someone in particular. I just wondered how you orient to the rage you're experiencing at this time in your life?

Heather: I mean, in general, my fuse is…I'll just say I've always had a short fuse with my redhead thing. So it was already short, and now it is literally like the bottom of the candle wick. For example, if anyone is incompetent or doesn't do their work–I get mad. I work so hard and try to give so much. With a job, you may not like it, but you still should give 100%. When people don't, my fuse is so short that I blow up. That's how my rage is functioning right now. I feel like people don't want to work anymore, and they don't want to do certain things. That really is a trigger for me. Then there's rage from not being heard. I remember I was listening to NPR, and a male doctor was on. I can't remember his name because it was a conversation I caught at the end. It was so riveting that I literally pulled off the side of the road to listen. One thing he said was that women's health is severely underserved. I was shocked. Wow, a man is saying this. But it's so true. We are completely underserved. It's ridiculous. Aren't there more women in this world than men anyway?

Tricia: Yes. It astounds me. I am without words. We all are going to go through menopause. And just like Alexandra said, it wasn't until relatively recently that they actually started testing for women. Without research and treatment options, how could you know how it is for us?

Alexandra: Thank you all. I have what I think will be my final question. I want to be deeply respectful of what each of you has shared, so I'm not looking to spiritually bypass or sugar coat anything, or be a Pollyanna–please don't hear what I'm asking in that way. Insofar as you've each described what I will call really shitty experiences of menopause. If that shit were to function as compost, what is there, if anything, that you see is possible? Is there anything worthwhile for you? With the right support, with the right vision? Is there any way that this passage can deliver you to somewhere you want to be?

Of course, it would be nice to have a more efficient way to get there. For sure! But I don't have that to offer. I would if I could, but I don't. The point is, is there any place you see this leading to which is actually a place you'd be glad to land in?

Keiya: I like that question. Yes, yes, yes, I appreciate that so much because, having been in the shit with menopause, there's just so much about it! One of the things I didn't share was that I had this inkling that there was someone out there that could help me feel better. The person I was referred to was in California, so I got on a plane right away. I didn't even take time to look for someone else, even though I live in New York. I was just clear that I'm heading to California, and that's that. Granted, it was easy for me to get there. But what Tricia was saying about looking for good care, taking so much energy, and taking so much out of you, that's real. So when I found there was a possibility, a chance to feel better, I trusted my gut and went with it. I also continued to go to California when I needed to get my refills.

Anyway, I got a bit off track, so I'll get back to the point. Having been in the shit and having gone through all of the things that I needed to go through to heal, to grow, it's almost like a rebirth, if you will. I'm looking at this now as such a beautiful experience because now I will be able to live my life differently. Not like I did when I was in my twenties. But I've tapped into a new level of resilience. I've tapped into a new level of wisdom. I really feel like this passage, this journey, has invited me to become a fuller, more well-rounded person. Before, I was attached to being a certain weight and looking a certain way. Now I am able to be okay with the new way things are. I also now make time to take care of myself. I know that it's okay for me to slow down. And I'm going to find a new way to generate income in order to be more creative. In summary, I really feel it's enabled me to tap into beautiful aspects of myself that I probably wouldn't have accessed had I not gone through this. Thank you again for the question.

Tricia: I love it. I love you.

Alexandra: I'm so glad for you. It's amazing to witness your experience.

Tricia: Heather and Maggie, you're both in the thick of it. I hope that what you've just heard gives you some comfort about what's on the other side of this experience.

Alexandra: I'm curious, do either of you have a response to what Keiya shared, from "Fuck no" to any other response? I know your attention is on what it feels like for you to be living your life right now, and it's challenging. Even so, I'm interested to hear any response you'd want to share.

Heather: Yes, if I relate it to my divorce, I can see something good is possible. When I was in the thick of getting divorced, I couldn't imagine being on the other side of it because it was just so miserable. I thought it was the worst thing that could happen to me. That was ten years ago. Now, in hindsight, I see that I'm so much happier. I'm in a much better place. Thank goodness that happened! I wouldn't want to still be stuck in that marriage, so I'm glad I went through the divorce. That's the only thing that gives me hope that this might be like that. Right now, I am just in the muck and trying to get out of it.

Tricia: It's gonna be a lot less, Heather, I promise you. Especially after today.

Heather: Yes. There's one more thing I thought about when Tricia told me that she was doing this that I want to mention. This could be a really weird tangent, but maybe not.

When I was dating in my early forties, I met a lot of men who were coming out of relationships with women who were at least ten years older or more than I was. When they talked about their marriages, they didn't point blank say that their former partners were going through menopause, but listening to them and now looking back, that seems like what was going on. I've learned that menopause is a pivotal time when many marriages fail. And I don't know, but I wonder if men were more informed, if it might help them to be more compassionate. I really do think that there's a point where men stick with a woman through this and understand it, or it breaks the relationship.

Tricia: Thank you.

Alexandra: I've heard that too, and I want to second what you've said, Heather.

I hope that this conversation has made all of you feel heard, seen, and held, because you are each so remarkable. I'm so grateful for you. Thank you so much for sharing your stories and insights with us.

Tricia: Yes, yes. Something new and extraordinary is being created right now by us and through us. This is a conversation that belongs to every one of us as we speak and as we listen. So thank you all so much for participating. I love you.

chapter 14

THIS IS THE RITUAL

Alexandra: Okay, we've discussed so many of the challenges with menopause. How are we providing solutions?

Tricia: We're not. We are having a conversation and inviting our readers to do the same.

Alexandra: Understood.

The reality is that you and I are two women in our fifties having conversations about things that are meaningful to us. That includes the fact that we are in menopause, whether we are discussing it overtly or not.

We've certainly talked about trauma today without calling it that. We've talked about how, in the context of menopause, we anticipate the transition will be traumatic and that, sometimes, it's actually quite wonderful.

Tricia: If we think about the men and women hearing our voices as they read our words, including trans and non-binary individuals if they take all of this as an invitation to reframe menopause and see it differently, then I think we've done a good job. Frankly, I would love it if we could shift the idea of menopause from one of dread or ignorance to one of empowerment, possibility, and transformation. I also want to inspire people to connect with one another around their experiences, just as we are doing here.

Alexandra: Me too!! That is exactly what I want too.

I want to name that all three of the women who joined us (not Pat) described wanting to control their bodies, to make them obey in terms of getting rid of various symptoms and feeling as they did in their twenties. That feels very different from how you speak about how it has been for you, which I would characterize as you collaborating with your body. Based on what has emerged this weekend, I would say that menopause seems to function as an invitation to harmonize with one's body or suffer. That's obviously not the whole story. There are physiological realities, too, causing real, intense physical symptoms. Of course. But the totality of our conversation has me wondering what would happen if we started telling young women (as early as teenagers but certainly by thirty-five) that they can learn to live in their own bodies in a collaborative way. They can surrender to, and align with, the inevitable changes, and doing so is glorious. Yes, there can be discipline and intention when it comes to exercise, nutrition, and medication, but even so, our bodies are a playground for change. Our bodies are meant to be in flux; control, judgment, and resistance are not the path to a vibrant midlife.

That's my takeaway from our tiny, statistically insignificant study. I would go so far as to say a person's inability to live comfortably inside her own body may set her up for a confusing, painful, or disappointing menopausal journey.

Tricia: Oh, you're absolutely right. That really is the one big difference between our menopausal experiences and theirs. It's not a matter of being good or bad, right or wrong. It's not about blame. It's about a relationship to the true thing underneath the cultural definitions of beauty, success, wellness, and anything else that gets in the way of our own sovereignty.

Alexandra: Agreed. I'd like to leave that hanging and just say a few things about sex before we conclude. There is an unfortunate dichotomy between conventional medical care, which doesn't honor so many women's experiences and, as a general rule, isn't equipped to handle menopause (although there are many exceptions to this rule), and holistic treatments. Many holistic treatments are actually effective and helpful, but it is very hard to distinguish between the effective treatments and those advertised by companies taking advantage of a desperate market. When we include economic considerations, privilege, and other relevant factors, we end up with the treacherous landscape of medical care women try to navigate. The result is that many women lack treatment for their menopausal symptoms.

One example is vaginal dryness. When I hear about painful sex due to vaginal dryness, it breaks my heart. No one should be having sex with a dry vagina, which results in pain, and often bleeding. There are many ways to successfully address that which are both straightforward and effective.

To be blunt, I take a stand for great sex being possible at all ages. If that's not happening, and a woman wants it, education and support are needed (in the form of medication, books, podcasts, and/or intimacy coaching).

Tricia: Beautifully said.

You know, I think it's because I am so clear on who I am that I am able to fully embrace myself and be in love with all of who I am in this phase. I'm sure that will be true in every other phase of my life as well. Knowing who I am and loving myself is not related to particular circumstances. It's directly related to my identity and my purpose. Going back to what Pat said yesterday, I don't care what other people think. I don't care about bursting into flames and having a hot flash on stage or anything else. It's because I know my mission so clearly and am in alignment with, and in full acceptance of, this phase of life–so much so that I reached out to you about writing a book about it!

Alexandra: Ha! Indeed you did!

When we first discussed this collaboration, I imagined we would come up with some kind of solution, some kind of ritual or something that would be available for women and their partners to do in order for all of us to reclaim menopause.

Tricia: We have! This is it! We're doing it. This right here is the ritual. We are sitting here creating something meaningful, and it truly is a ritual born of sisterhood. Just as indigenous cultures honored rites of passage with ritual and meaningful experiences, we are birthing that for ourselves in our menopause passage through having this conversation.

This was never intended to be a book about solving anyone's menopause problems, once and for all. This is a book about having a conversation, inviting others to join us in the conversation, and inspiring readers to start their own as well. I think that's really, really important. If we can communicate that, it will be empowering. Conversations are a beginning. They remove some of the loneliness and isolation. They can break down the taboos in the culture which otherwise strangle us. If we remember, this book is literally a conversation that happened between us and a few other people over the course of two days. Just imagine what's possible for every woman who wants to participate for a few minutes or for a few months or years, as her experience evolves. That's what this is. Nothing more, nothing less.

I feel so fulfilled and nourished. I knew I would feel this way, but I didn't know just how deeply fulfilling and nourishing I would find it.

Alexandra: Yes. Me too.

Tricia: And again, I want to express gratitude for our choosing to walk into the unknown together, for being right here, right now, and also for what having done this means for each of us for the rest of our lives.

Alexandra: Me too. I'm so grateful–for your inspiration and for each moment in our extended conversation.

Tricia: We both walked into the unknown and came out on the other side.

Alexandra: We did, we did. Together.

Tricia: I love you.

Alexandra: I love you too.

Tricia: We are complete.

ACKNOWLEDGMENTS

We could not have created this book without the genius of Barrie Cole. She helped us shape the container and turned the transcripts into something artful and compelling. She understood our intention and both honored and contributed to our vision; we are very grateful.

We are also grateful to Pat Ducksworth, Heather, Keiya and Maggie for sharing their lived experiences and thoughtful reflections with us. Thank you for being in the sisterhood.

We also want to acknowledge our husbands, Joe Ricci and Rodd Stockwell, for their support throughout this process.

ABOUT THE AUTHORS

With over thirty years of experience in film, TV, and theater, Tricia Brouk uses her platform to create a safe, inclusive space for others to use their influential voices for impact. She has put thousands of speakers onto big stages and is the Founder of The Big Talk Academy. *The Invitation* is another way for her to contribute to the bigger conversation and remind you that you are not alone. When we begin to talk about what every woman goes through with compassion, truth, and acceptance, we can empower women and men everywhere. www.triciabrouk.com

Known as "The Intimacy Doctor," Alexandra Stockwell, MD, is a Relationship and Intimacy Coach and an Intimate Marriage Expert who specializes in coaching ambitious, successful couples to build beautiful, long-lasting, passionate relationships. For over 20 years, she has shown men and women how to bring pleasure and purpose into all aspects of life: from the daily grind of running a household to intimate communication and ecstatic experiences in the bedroom. Her mission is to change the cultural narrative so people everywhere know that intimate relationships can flourish and improve with time. www.alexandrastockwell.com

When Tricia and Alexandra call one another, they pick up. Their conversations are deep, significant, and fun, as is this book.

www.ingramcontent.com/pod-product-compliance
Lightning Source LLC
Chambersburg PA
CBHW022050020426
42335CB00012B/632